Dancing with Alzheimer's

Dancing with Alzheimer's

Revised Edition

Dolores Attias

iUniverse, Inc.
New York Lincoln Shanghai

Dancing with Alzheimer's

iUniverse books may be ordered through booksellers or by contacting:

iUniverse
2021 Pine Lake Road, Suite 100
Lincoln, NE 68512
www.iuniverse.com
1-800-Authors (1-800-288-4677)

Front cover by Japhlet Bire Attias and the iUniverse design team.

ISBN-13: 978-0-595-37351-2 (pbk)
ISBN-13: 978-0-595-67488-6 (cloth)
ISBN-13: 978-0-595-81748-1 (ebk)
ISBN-10: 0-595-37351-8 (pbk)
ISBN-10: 0-595-67488-7 (cloth)
ISBN-10: 0-595-81748-3 (ebk)

Printed in the United States of America

To my late sister Alma for her encouragement and feedback any time I asked for it, and to my brother Eddy who parted without seeing my book. My eternal thanks to my dearest Maria Elena Ramirez Cabañas for everything she has done for me.

Contents

Acknowledgments

Deep thanks to my friends and family for their help.

My children: Miriam, Messod and Setty Attias. My grandchildren: Setty Margarita Magana and Japhlet Bire Attias. My friends: Lola Walker and Sue Millard who proof read Dancing with Alzheimer's many times. Special thanks to Doctor Rafael Magana and Barbara Harrington, who believed in me and donated hours of her precious time.

My gratitude for all the help I received from my writers group, Pinellas Authors and Writers Organization (PINAWOR).

1

Meeting Mrs. Bromley

I stood on Sand Key Bridge gazing into the Tampa Bay waters, which today were unusually rough; hair blew in my face and I brushed it away from my eyes. The violently crashing waves paralleled my inner turmoil and sense of desperation. Was there no way out? Scanning the foam formed by the receding waves, I saw a collage of images from my life. In the past I was always laughing, entertaining, wearing expensive clothes, surrounded by beautiful people; the personification of happiness. Was I happy?

Mauricio had constantly reminded me that I owed him everything; that he had secured for me a heavenly bliss, that I was the envy of our acquaintances, and with good reason: He was young, virile, handsome, wealthy, and kept me as a queen. Why hadn't I been happy then? I had no money problems, and according to him, I was sexually satisfied. I had three healthy and wonderful children, whom the governess and nannies attended to, freeing me from sleepless nights and the pressures of their upbringing.

He took care of everything that money could buy, but he had never been able to buy me my own identity. *His* identity was more than enough for the both of us. I had been empty and had lived a life with no purpose. For too long I had been his shadow, and shadows cannot be happy. When his obsession for power suffocated me, I fled the golden cage and escaped to Miami. After a painful separation I managed to get the down payment for a house and a generous monthly allowance but I lost my children, which stabbed me like a dagger in my heart. Through time his help dwindled and I was forced to sell my jewelry and other valuables to pay bills and make mortgage payments. Eventually, there was nothing of value left to sell and now I was about to lose my home.

My children were already grown up and although we had a very close relationship, they had their own life to live far away from me. I felt lonely and desperate. My usual optimism had deserted me. I recalled Scarlet O'Hara's last words in *Gone with the Wind*: "I'll think about it tomorrow." But I was afraid that this time, there was no tomorrow for me. I couldn't hold back the tears any longer, so I let them run freely. Although there was no one around, I felt self-conscious, so I hurried back home to be alone with my sadness and my prayers.

Once home, I splashed cold water on my face and struggled to restrain the tears—as though stopping the tears would halt the pain in my heart. The journey to the past had drained me. I felt defeated, lost and disoriented.

The ringing of the phone startled me. I fought to collect my emotions and reluctantly picked up the receiver.

"Hello?" I mumbled.

"Hi, Lolita. Is that you?"

It was my good friend Hugh.

"Oh hi, Hugh."

"Are you all right?" He sounded concerned.

"Yes, Hugh, I'm fine, thank you,"

"You sure don't sound it, but anyhow, I have some good news. At least, I think it's good news," he said enthusiastically. "I found the ideal job for you!"

"A job? You mean a paying job?" I asked incredulously. "You wouldn't be kidding, would you?"

"No. I'm not kidding. And it pays very, very well. Are you interested?"

"Yes, I'm interested," I responded quickly. "But what kind of a job is it?" I was skeptical; I had no work experience and I had always had people do everything for me. Would I be able to hold a job?

"I believe that this is a job with your name written on it."

"Really?"

"How would you like to drive a rich, old British lady around town, take her shopping, and eat at the best restaurants in the Bay Area every day?" Hugh asked, with amusement in his voice.

Everything sounded so good, I thought. In fact, too good. God let it be true…I was speechless.

"Hello? Are you still there? Lolita?"

"Yes, Hugh, I'm still here. That job sounds too good to be true. What else would I have to do?"

He laughed. "Just what I told you; believe me."

"There must be a catch."

"No catch. A friend of mine is looking for a companion for his eighty-eight-year-old grandmother. I told him about you, and that you were perfect for the job."

"Thanks for your vote of confidence." I paused for a second. "Is there something wrong with the old lady?"

"She's as healthy as a horse."

"Then why does she need a full-time companion?"

"She's in the early stages of Alzheimer's. Consequently, she's forgetful, but other than that, she's okay."

"But I don't know anything about Alzheimer's," I confessed.

"Don't worry. You're going to be her companion, not her nurse; she doesn't need one yet. Oh, and there's no housework involved."

"Still, Hugh, she must need some special care."

"Nothing of the sort. Keep her company and help her remember that she prefers Neiman Marcus to Bloomingdale's and duck *à l'orange* over caviar—that's all. She could remain in this stage for a long time. Mrs. Bromley has had an interesting life as a performer on the Paris stage. You'll enjoy her wit."

"Oh, Hugh, you have no idea how important this is to me, and how much I need a job, especially now." I cleared my throat and continued; "The answer is definitely yes!"

I hung up the phone. Could this be the answer to my prayers?

Later that evening, I thought about the bills that were piling up and the stress of my financial burden. I couldn't get my problems off my mind. God only knew how I'd meet my monthly tally. I walked to the window and searched the heavens for a sign from my guardian angel, which had always come to my rescue. When I saw a bright star that seemed to wink at me, I took it as a sign, the sign I needed. I don't know how long I stood there, but eventually I felt divine inner harmony and strength. Cuddled in my dreamy mood, I welcomed the feelings of peace that this turn of events had engendered in my being.

Full of expectation, I waited until the new day arrived.

The next morning, I woke up earlier than usual. I was nervous and anxious to meet Mr. Williams, the woman's grandson. I drove along Gulf Boulevard as if for the first time, through numerous animated beach towns, alongside cafes with people sitting on the patios having breakfast. The scene reminded me of Madrid in my well-to-do times, when I took money for granted. I wished I could hold in my hand a fraction of the money I had spent so inconsequentially. My attention returned to the road, where colorful boutiques, luxury hotels, and exotic restaurants dressed up the quaint towns.

When I saw the landmark, the Don Cesar pink hotel, I turned left and crossed a causeway flanked by a spectacular view of Boca Ciega Bay. Different hues of blue covered the vast sky, which was spotted with white, cotton-like clouds. An array of waterfront mansions displayed stunning landscapes. The lush greenery of the panorama caught my attention; this exclusive neighborhood somehow had being spared from the drought and the strict watering laws, which were enforced in this part of Florida.

I finally arrived at my destination. I felt my stomach flutter, and took a deep breath as I reached for a mirror to check my makeup. *I must look my best for this, the first job interview in my life.* I parked in front of the house, which was surrounded by a white wrought-iron fence. I sent a prayer to *La Virgen de la Caridad* and rang the bell.

A handsome young man welcomed me at the door. His smile exposed even white teeth that contrasted with his tanned face. His blue jeans and snug white T-shirt revealed an athletic body.

"I'm Gary Williams," he said extending his hand. "And you must be Dolores Rimblas. I'm very glad to meet you."

"Thank you; me too. And please, call me Lolita."

"Lolita Rimblas," he said, smiling.

I followed him into a spacious living room, decorated with African motifs. A lion's head baring huge fangs hovered over the far end of a wall.

"Sit down, please." He pointed to the couch and sat across from me. "Did you have any problems finding the house?"

"Not at all."

"Good. Well, let's not waste any time and get started. I don't need any references—Hugh spoke highly of you and told me a little bit about your life." He smiled. "My only reservation is that you might, eventually, get tired of my grandmother's constant repetition and forgetfulness."

"I don't think I will. I'm a very patient person. I was married to a very demanding man."

"Hugh told me about it. That's why we thought you were the right person to deal with my grandmother. Besides being forgetful, she is…how should I put this…difficult."

My heart skipped a beat, as Mr. Williams continued.

"We pay one hundred dollars a shift to ensure that my grandmother is well taken care of. We have a cleaning service, so your only obligation is attending to her. There's very little cooking involved. She eats lunch out every day, and sometimes dinner too." He laughed. "My grandmother is never too tired or sick to go to a restaurant. Now, I'll be happy to answer any questions you may have."

I pondered for a moment and asked, "Who pays for the food?"

"My grandmother does. With certain restrictions, she still manages her checkbook. It amuses her to go to the bank and to the grocery store. It makes her happy to buy tons of makeup and beauty products that she doesn't need, but there's nothing we can do about that," he said, laughing. Then he asked, "Is there anything else you would like to know?"

"What are my hours going to be?"

"Well, your shift runs from about six in the afternoon to seven-thirty in the morning."

The news came as a shock. I had assumed it would be in the daytime. I struggled to find my voice. "I'm confused, Mr. Williams. Hugh didn't mention that I would have to spend the night here."

"Oh no! I'm so sorry, but that's when we need you."

"Well, then, do you think that I may have a chance for the day shift later on?"

"I'm sorry, Miss Rimblas, but I doubt it. We have a woman who's been with us for a long time, and she takes care of my grandmother during the day." He paused for a moment. "Is that going to be a problem?"

"No," I said, forcing a smile.

"Good. Let me tell you more about my grandmother. She lives right next door to me, which is very convenient." He grimaced. "Please let me be very candid Miss Rimblas, my grandmother not only repeats the same things over and over, but she has a terrible temper, and her moods change constantly. It's been hard finding someone willing to put up with her."

"Are you trying to discourage me?" I asked.

"No. I need you desperately, but I want to be fair." He ran his fingers through his hair. "I just want you to be prepared when you meet her because if she doesn't like something about you, she'll say it to your face. You never know what she'll come up with next. But I'm sure it will work out." He scratched his chin. "You should have no problem with her. She likes smart, classy people."

"Thank you. I'll try to live up to your expectations."

"And if you take the job, I'll back you all the way." He stood up. "Just one more thing, Miss Rimblas: can you start tomorrow?"

Although I was delighted to start earning an income, I still resented the misunderstanding about the hours. My resentment turned into resignation swiftly and I nodded automatically.

Mr. Williams looked at me and raised an eyebrow. "Is that a yes?"

"Of course—yes," I answered quickly.

"Great. Then let's go meet her now."

I followed him through a tastefully decorated dining room with a mirrored wall, then to an enclosed back porch with several scattered baby toys. We walked through an outside wet bar surrounded by palm trees and hibiscus plants in full bloom. The briny scent from Boca Ciega Bay floated through the air. As we strolled along the well-manicured garden, I admired the colorful rose beds, palm trees, shrubbery, and various marble statues lining the way. The lawn looked inviting, the lawn chairs even more so. Mr. Williams stopped at the rear of a two story house and turned to me.

"This is her home," he said, signaling toward the house.

I followed him into the living room, which had a cathedral-dome ceiling and stained-glass windows.

"*Grandmere! grandmere!*" Mr. Williams called out in French. "Poor soul, she's hard of hearing. We have to constantly remind her to wear her hearing aids." He walked over to a stairway and called again, "*Grandmere!*"

I went over to the far wall to admire a magnificent, huge painting of a handsome, middle-aged lady with expressive, deep-blue eyes. A striking diamond and sapphire necklace embellished her swan-like neck. Then…I saw it…an incredible life-size statue of a woman. She had extended arms, reaching to the ceiling, unconcerned about her nudity.

"That's my grandmother," Mr. Williams said, with a tinge of nostalgia in his voice. "She was a beauty."

Suddenly a high-pitched voice seemed to fill the room. "Darling, what are you doing here so early?"

I turned toward the voice and was impressed to see a tall, elegant lady addressing Mr. Williams.

"Come, my darling," she said as she extended her hands to him.

Then, turning sharply, she glanced at me. "And who is this?"

"This is Lolita. She's going to be your night companion."

"Who? Speak clearly, Gary. Who is this person?"

He looked at me apologetically. "Please, *grandmere*, watch your manners!"

"Well, then, who is she?"

"Lolita Rimblas."

"Who?"

"Lo-li-ta," he said slowly.

"What?"

"Lo-li-ta!" he shouted.

She frowned. "Lopeta?"

"Lolita," I said timidly. "My name is Lolita."

"Pleeease *grandmere*," Mr. Williams pleaded, "go get your hearing aids."

With the posture of a queen, she waltzed out of the room, leaving behind the trail of a soft perfume that contradicted her hard personality.

Right away I didn't like the snobbish woman. A chill ran down my spine when I realized my situation: I was going to work for this woman—be her companion for hours each day. I need, by all means, to be humble to be able to overcome her haughtiness. *O God, help me!* I prayed, while admiring a beautiful painting.

"That's a limited edition print of Cézanne's Bathers," Mr. Williams said as he pointed to the painting. "My grandmother has a large collection of drawings and oils. We keep some originals under lock."

He went over to a black lacquered cabinet filled with jade figurines; most of them were dogs with sparkling diamond eyes.

"She's crazy about dogs," Mr. Williams continued. "You'll find that out soon enough."

"What will she find out soon?" Mrs. Bromley said as she returned. "Now tell me again who this woman is."

"This is Lolita." He sighed.

"What is she doing here?"

"She's going to be your night companion."

"My what?"

He shook his head. "Lolita will be staying with you at night, so you're not alone when Molly leaves."

"Hmm. *Bon*. I suppose it's better than nothing."

This woman has no tact at all. Her remark both surprised and offended me.

"Sorry, Lolita," Mr. Williams quickly said. "I warned you that she says whatever comes to mind without thinking."

"There's no need to apologize for me," Mrs. Bromley stated in a piercing voice.

Although I was hurt, I did my best to hide it. "I understand, Mr. Williams," I said. "Don't worry about it."

He looked relieved and patted my shoulder. "Good. I'm very glad you understand."

Then he turned to his grandmother. "*Grandmere*, it is time for your program." He handed her the TV remote and gestured for me to follow him. "Come on, Lolita. I'd like you to meet Molly. She's our right hand."

"Good-bye, Mrs. Bromley," I said. "I'm looking forward to seeing you again tomorrow."

"Too bad I can't say the same," she said as she sat in front of the television set and started flipping channels.

When we were in the vestibule, I said, "I'm afraid she doesn't like me, Mr. Williams."

"I understand that her rudeness makes you think so, but if she had disliked you she would have told you so in no uncertain ways."

"But, isn't that what she did?"

"No Lolita, I think she accepted you." Mr. Williams said with a warm smile.

A petite, middle-aged brunette walked in, carrying a miniature salt-and-pepper schnauzer.

"Molly, this is Lolita. She's going to do the night shift," Mr. Williams said. Molly smiled, placed the dog on the floor, and shook my hand. "Nice to meet you."

Mr. Williams flashed a playful grin. "I know that both of you will take good care of my grandmother," he said. "And Lolita, if you run into trouble, Molly is the one to call."

I was wondering why I should contact Molly instead of him when I felt the dog jump on my legs and his shrill bark startled me. Molly pulled the dog away.

"Bowdie is welcoming you. This little rascal is all bark and no bite," she said.

"This dog is a very important part of my grandmother's life," Mr. Williams added. "And if you want to win her over, make a lot of fuss about her little girl."

I patted the dog's head. "Is she a puppy?"

"Hardly," Molly exclaimed. "She's thirteen. That's around ninety in people years."

"Oh, my word," I said, "she's in pretty good shape for her age."

Molly laughed. "Yeah, I wish I could say the same for myself."

On my way home, I pondered. I liked Mr. Williams. I liked Molly. I even liked Bowdie. But Elizabeth Bromley…?

That evening I took a warm bath, wrapped myself in a bathrobe, and curled up in bed to call my sister-in-law, Minerva, who lived in Miami. She was married to my brother Eddy, and the three of us were very close. I wanted to share my good news with them.

"That's wonderful," said Minerva when I told her about the job. "You sound enthusiastic, but the woman sounds nuts. I hope your dream job doesn't turn into a nightmare."

I don't know why people always expect the worst. A little cross, I answered, "Being pessimistic never helps. We have to always expect the best."

"I'm practical, Lolita. And by all means, don't take this as a bad omen."

"Then don't say it, for heaven's sake! Don't rain on my party," I said, troubled.

"Excuse me, *por favor*. I'm only trying to prepare you," she apologized.

I felt badly. "I'm sorry I barked at you. I'm tense. I'm thrilled and petrified at the same time...I don't want anything to go wrong. The money sounds great, but I'm disappointed about not getting the day shift." I glanced around sadly at all my belongings, not knowing if I was going to be able to save them. "I hate sleeping away from home, but we can't have it all, can we? I'll just make my room cozy over there."

"If I know you," Minerva said, "you'll make the best of the situation."

"Better still, since I won't be using my bedroom and I need the money to pay off my debts, I figure I might as well rent it, and—"

"Wait," she interrupted. "Not so fast. What if things don't work out? What if she doesn't like you?"

"I'll do my best to make her like me. This is going to work if it's the last thing I do."

"Please Lolita, don't rush things. Wait until you're sure the job is yours. Maybe you can't stomach her."

Although I was annoyed at Minerva's negativity, I said. "I'm in no position to be picky, Minerva. Besides, most of the time she'll be sleeping. That's the only good thing about the night hours. I won't see much of her."

"Listen to me," Minerva said patiently. "I'm not saying it's not going to work or that you should not rent out your room, all I'm asking you to do is to wait for a few weeks to be sure everything works out. In the mean time you can rent any of the other rooms in the house."

"Okay, I promise I'll keep my room for now." I said, thinking that Minerva made sense.

"I'm happy to hear you say that."

"Oh, Minerva, I can't wait until I see my first pay check. It'll be the first money I've ever earned in my life. Can you believe that? Almost seventy years old and I'm starting my first job!"

"I'm proud of you Lolita, and more so because it's the first time I hear you telling your real age."

"I don't see the point on trying to hide my age any more. I thank God for this opportunity, and I'm planning to be the best companion this woman has ever had. And I will be!"

"I know you will work hard," she said. Then she added with authority, "I know the money is good, but I'm afraid every penny will cost you dearly."

"Stop, please! Have mercy!" I laughed. "I'm going to sleep now; I have a big day tomorrow. *Buenas noches.*"

"*Por favor*, Lolita. Keep me posted. *Buenas noches y buena suerte.*"

2

Paris Match

"Welcome, dear. Come on in," Mrs. Bromley said sweetly standing at the doorway, smiling. "Molly had an appointment and couldn't wait for you." I was surprised to be greeted so pleasantly. After her rudeness at our first meeting, I had expected more of the same.

"I'm sorry, Mrs. Bromley. Am I late?" I asked as I stepped inside.

"Not at all. I'll take you around and show you my home. Bowdie," she called, "come on! Come with Mommy."

I placed my overnight case in the vestibule and followed her as she proceeded to give me a tour of the house.

"As you can see," she said, "my house is filled with mementos from my past and my trips abroad."

With amazing agility, she climbed the stairs that led to a parlor furnished with a contemporary green leather sofa that contrasted with an antique rollup desk.

"What's your name?" she asked, turning to face me.

"Lolita. My name is Lolita Rimblas."

She pointed at two doors, stopped at one of them, faced me and asked, "What's your name, dear?"

"Lo-li-ta," I enunciated as clearly as I could.

"Oh yes, Lopeta, those rooms are forbidden, so keep away from them. Jane is the only one with the keys. Only God knows what she hides there. One day I'll force her to open them for me. After all, this is my house, and I pay for everything. Jane has no right to take over my house. I'm warning you: keep away from her." She became more agitated and I wondered who Jane was and why Mrs. Bromley had warned me about her. I found it very odd. She continued to the end of the hall and opened the last door. The ceiling fan was on, wafting an aroma of lavender that I perceived as welcoming.

"This is the Jacuzzi," she said, entering the room. "And that's an electric chaise lounge; it massages you automatically. I don't use it anymore."

I wanted to ask if I could use it, but I changed my mind.

"How do you like my paintings?" she asked pointing to a cadre of oil paintings.

"You painted them?" I kidded.

"No, you idiot. Can't you recognize Mary Cassat?"

Her insult hit me like a ton of bricks. I was just trying to humor her and she called me an idiot.

"This other one," she said, entering another room, "is filled with figurines I collected from diverse parts of the world."

I was in awe admiring the vast collection of porcelain, ceramic, marble, and bronze figurines. I felt as if I were at an exhibition of antiques. "This is wonderful. I could spend hours here," I said truthfully.

"But you can't right now," she said, with a cute smile. Then abruptly added, "Let's go to the kitchen."

As I followed her, I wondered about Jane and whether there really was a secret behind those doors. The way she had spoken about Jane showed resentment, and I wonder why.

Once in the kitchen, she took a paper bag from the refrigerator and handed it to me. "It's a rotisserie chicken from Publix. I suggest you use your creativity and fix us a gourmet dinner. Make sure you never use onions. I'm deathly allergic to them"

"A gourmet dinner?" I whispered incredulously.

"Did you say something?"

"No. I didn't say anything."

"What did you say?"

"I didn't say anything, Mrs. Bromley."

"*Bon*! Now it is teatime and later drinks before supper. Feel at home and eat anything you want. I want you to write down a list of what you like, and Molly and I will shop tomorrow." Suddenly she rushed out of the kitchen, calling for Molly.

I walked after her into the living room. "Molly isn't here," I explained.

"I know that. I'm calling you. Don't you know who you are?'

"Yes, I do. I am Lolita," I said.

"Molly? Lopeta? Lolita? What bloody difference does it make? If Molly isn't here, who do you suppose I'm calling?"

"Me," I managed to say. "But you don't have to be rude to me."

"It's more fun. It amuses me."

"Kindness works better," I replied.

"But it is predictable and boring," she snapped back. "Molly, you don't have any sense of humor—no wit at all."

I felt attacked and mocked. I thought it would be best if I retreated to the kitchen in order to avoid a confrontation. "I'm going to prepare your tea, Mrs. Bromley," I said smiling. "Would you excuse me, please?"

"Come back here!" she ordered as I started for the door. "That can wait. Sit down and tell me about yourself. I still need to find out if I like you." She stared at me and I felt how her gaze penetrated me. "Do you have a family? Are you married? Is there a man in your life?"

"I'm divorced," I said

"What did you say?"

"I'm divorced," I repeated, raising my voice.

"Don't just stand there. Have a seat."

I sat down on the nearest chair and was about to relax when she screamed, "Get off that chair! Can't you see it's a Louis XVI antique, a priceless piece and very delicate?"

I jumped up. "Where would you like me to sit, then?"

"Anywhere you want. Just don't break anything," she said as she picked up the shaggy dog and placed it on the antique chair. "Look at her, Molly. She looks like a queen."

I looked around and sat on the couch. *God help me. I'm going to need more patience than I thought.*

"Do you have a degree on something? In what?"

"I didn't know I needed a degree to work as a companion."

"It's not required, but it would help me decide if I like you or not."

That was all I needed. A PhD in patience would come handy right about now. I mulled that over for a few moments.

"Do you have one?" Mrs. Bromley insisted.

"No. I don't," I confessed embarrassed.

"What did you say? Speak up! You mumble all the time!"

"No, I do not," I repeated.

"I'm sure you will find a way to make up for it. Do you have children? How many?" She sat next to me.

"I have a son and a daughter who live in Mexico. My oldest daughter lives in Minnesota."

"Do you live alone?"

"Yes, I do."

"Do you have a boyfriend?"

"No, I don't."

"You don't have to lie. Is he rich?"

I took a deep breath and said, "I don't have one."

"A beauty like you? Are you a lesbian?"

"Of course not!" I snapped in shock.

"Why are you so shocked? There is nothing wrong with liking someone of the same sex, you know?" She smiled mischievously. "Don't you need a man? How old are you?"

"Well…" I hesitated, "I am…seventy," I confessed painfully. There, I did it. For the second time I told my age.

She threw her head back and laughed, showing her own, even, white teeth. "Are you that old? Oh my! A very young seventy, you look fifty! Just like me. I am fifty, I think, but I have been told that I look much younger. What do you think?" before I could answer she continued, "I don't have a man because my brilliant late husband Robert, left our estate in Jupiter Island to his daughter. Millionaires are a dime a dozen there, and I'm sure that if I had stayed there, I would have married any one of them. Sneaky Robert! I'm sure he did it on purpose, and now my family keeps me under watch. I can't even remember the last time I had sex."

She leaned over, reached for a trunk next to a sliding glass door, and took out a huge scrapbook. Given the obvious weight of the album, I was impressed that an eighty-eight-year-old person could lift it so effortlessly.

Mrs. Bromley began turning pages as she explained the photographs and clips that were her history.

"I was only one in this picture," she said, handing me a photo. "That's how I learned to walk, by holding on to my dog's tail. We vacationed on the beach in Bristol. I mean Bristol, England, not Rhode Island."

"I didn't know there was a Bristol in the United States," I said.

"Well, now you know."

I looked at the photo of a pretty girl embracing a handsome collie. "Oh, how beautiful," I said, handing it back to her.

"Did you say something?" she asked.

"I just said how beautiful," I repeated.

"In this one with my father, I was twelve," she went on. "He used to hit my shoulders with a stick if I didn't sit upright and demanded that I always have proper posture."

"So that's why you keep your back so straight," I said.

"Yes." She handed me another. "See? This is Zinna, my older sister. We were both dancers. This picture was taken when we performed in Paris. We replaced the Dolly Sisters in the Moulin Rouge. When Zinna married a millionaire, I joined the Can-Can, I remember like it was yesterday when I joined *La Revue des Folies Bergere*.

You know, my sister was bosom buddies with the queen of Spain." She laughed and rubbed her index and middle fingers together. No funny stuff, you know."

"Really?" I replied.

"Are you calling me a liar?" she snapped indignantly.

"Of course not." I wasn't sure what she was insinuating, but I quickly searched for an explanation and came out with, "I am just very impressed."

"Bon," to my relief, she continued. "And look at this one. This is my only son from my second husband." The picture depicted a hospital room and a young Mrs. Bromley with her hair in an attractive chignon, holding a newborn baby on her lap. "This baby was an accident because I didn't like children and never planned on having any. I had a perfect figure and didn't want to spoil it for anything in the world. This other one is with the baby's nurse holding him as we all left the hospital."

In one newspaper clipping yellowed by age, a handsome man was seated next to her. She explained, "My husband was a movie star, besieged by women, no matter where we went. I didn't know that women threw themselves so shamelessly at men. Women pulled him away from me in the streets, and although they didn't look like prostitutes, they acted like them."

There were more newspaper clippings with photos of herself and her husband at social events. The *Paris Match* showed her wearing a fur coat and holding the leash of an Afghan hound. Dozens more photos appeared in other magazines, all with large, purebred dogs.

"Do you like dogs?" she asked as she closed the album and placed it back in the trunk.

For a moment I didn't answer. I wanted to be sincere. I liked dogs, just not in the house. It bothered me to see them jumping on people, wagging their tails and knocking down precious figurines.

"I'm waiting," Mrs. Bromley said harshly. "Do you like dogs or not?"

I remembered Mr. Williams's advice: *If you want to win her over, make a fuss about Bowdie*. "I love dogs," I finally said.

"What did you say?"

"I said I love dogs."

"It certainly took you forever to answer."

Bowdie was sleeping on the antique chair. She picked it up, then sat next to me on the couch, and placed the dog between us. "Get acquainted with my treasure. Go on, say something meaningful to my baby."

I racked my brain trying to think of something meaningful to say to a dog. "Hi, baby," I ventured. "How are you doing? You're so cute." I felt silly but couldn't find anything clever to say, so I patted its head.

"When I was mugged in Paris," she said, clutching the dog, "this little treasure saved my life. I owe her. Yes, I do." She kissed the dog, which in turn licked her entire face for what to me seemed an eternity. "Now it's your turn, Molly. Kiss Bowdie."

Me kiss an animal? God forbid!

Suddenly, she got up.

"Oh, Lord," she exclaimed. "Look at the time. We'll skip tea today, it's time for my drinkypoo."

Saved by her drinky-poo, whatever that was. I followed her to the wet bar, where she took out a huge bottle of whiskey and put ice in two glasses.

"Keep this in mind: scotch with ginger ale at six every day. Do you understand? Now, have a drink with me, Molly."

Her persistence on calling me Molly shouldn't bother me, but it reminded me of years past when I had no identity. "If you don't mind," I said softly, "would you be kind enough to call me by my name? I'm Lolita."

"So what? Lolita or Molly or Ginger—who cares? Drink with me."

"I don't drink."

"Don't be a bore. Drink up!" she ordered.

What's the point in arguing? I took a sip, then another, followed by another, everything in the room started to spin.

"Not so fast, Molly, it isn't water! Enjoy it sip by sip." Her expression softened. She laughed, and I laughed with her. She beckoned. "Come to my bedroom."

Her bedroom? What in the world did she want me to go to her bedroom for? Hesitantly, I followed.

On the tour of the house earlier, she had pointed out her bedroom from the hall. Now, once inside, I noticed a black mink bedspread covered with stuffed animals. It could have been a child's room if it hadn't been for a stand holding a bottle of liqueur at the foot of the bed. I hoped she didn't drink at night; I didn't need to take care of a person with a drinking problem. It really worried me.

"Let's put my babies away," she said, clearing the bed. "Take note. This is part of our routine." She unfolded the sheet and placed her negligee and a bar of Toblerone chocolate on one corner.

It annoyed me that I was faltering, but after a few deep breaths, I felt steadier. I would make sure not to drink that much again.

After dinner we watched *Wheel of Fortune*, and I was surprised at her accuracy and grasp of the rules of the game. My wonder increased when she answered still more difficult questions from *Jeopardy*. I found it amazing that in spite of her age and Alzheimer's, she was able to bring the knowledge from her past to the uncertainty of her present.

She turned the TV off, and I brought in her pills, as Molly had instructed.

"What are these?" she yelled.

"Your nightly pills."

"What are you talking about?"

"Your pills."

"Are you trying to kill me?"

I was startled. How could her demeanor change so quickly? One minute she was sweet and laughing, and the next she was accusing me of trying to murder her. I did not think she was joking.

"Hey, I'm talking to you," she said, pointing a finger in my face. "What are these bloody pills for?"

Molly should have explained what the damned pills were for. I never thought to ask.

"I asked you what they are!"

I knew I had to say something, so I held out the pills. "This one is for your blood pressure, the pink tiny one is for your heart, this one helps you sleep, and this one is for your brain."

"Where's the one for the bathroom? That's the one I need the most."

I pointed to the pink one. "That one right there."

"Are you sure? You said that one was for my heart."

She caught me unprepared, so I ventured. "Well, it's a laxative too."

"Swear."

"Yes, I swear," I replied crossing my fingers. I felt awful.

"You swear? Is that what you said? You are mumbling."

"I swear."

"*Bon*," she said, and swallowed all of them.

"Will you need any help?"

"From you?" she snapped. "You're no help at all!"

I went to my bedroom and closed the door. Moments later I heard a knock.

"I want to talk with you immediately," Mrs. Bromley said as she opened the door and entered the room, followed by the dog.

"Is something wrong?" I asked.

"I never want your door closed."

I started to protest. "Why does my door have to be—?"

"Bowdie and I want to have access to your room in case of an emergency," she interrupted.

"But Mrs. Bromley, you can call me on the intercom anytime."

"Don't try to be smart. Bowdie can't use the intercom, so good night and sweet dreams."

After she left I got into bed, but could not fall asleep with the door wide open. The house was strange to me, and I felt nervous and uneasy. Later, between exhaustion and the comfort of a feather mattress, I eventually fell into a deep sleep, only to be awakened by a blinding light in my face. For a moment I didn't know where I was. My heart was pounding. Terrified, I placed my hands in front of my eyes. "Who's there?" I screamed.

"It is me, Molly. Who else would it be?" She laughed loudly and moved the light away from me. "Did you think it was your lover?"

I saw her shadowy figure hovering over me, with two flashlights just inches away from my face.

"For God's sake, what are you doing?" I cried out.

"Are you okay, my darling?"

"I was, until you scared me half to death."

She started out the door, hesitated, and then turned on the light. "You should thank me for caring. Some people are ungrateful. I only wanted to make sure you were still alive." She shut the light off and walked away. "So much fuss for nothing. Let's get out of here, Bowdie."

There was no chance of a restful night now. I left the night-light on, since the darkness played tricks on me. Questions about her sanity plagued me, and I wondered if she was violent. I hadn't seen a knife in her hand, but one could have been hidden. Maybe that's why she wanted the door left open. I wondered if I should keep a job with such an unpredictable and irascible person. I was told that the only problem was her loss of memory. Loss of memory my...No money in the world was worth losing my sanity. *Virgen de la Caridad*, protect me.

I was wide-awake when the first rays of sun crept into the room. Soon after, I heard the shuffle of feet coming toward my room. I cringed.

Suddenly, Mrs. Bromley was at the door. "May I come in?"

She came in before I could answer, carrying a tray with a cup of coffee, a newspaper, and a withered red rose on top of a linen napkin. To make the scene complete, the dog walked in after her.

"Good morning, darling. I hope you slept well."

As angry as I had been, I was moved by her thoughtfulness. I concluded that I had made a storm out of a glass of water. It touched me that she had brought me coffee—even if it was black and bitter—and the withered rose added a nice touch. My anger waned.

"Very kind of you, Mrs. Bromley. Thank you."

While dressing, I forced myself to think positively. I was humming *Ode to Joy*, one of my favorite melodies, when Mrs. Bromley stormed into my room and started emptying drawers and throwing pillows to the floor.

"May I help you, Mrs. Bromley?

"Shut up. They must be under the padding," she said.

"What in the world are you looking for?"

"Where are you hiding my papers?"

"What papers?"

"The ones with the stories about my colleagues."

"I don't know what you are talking about, Mrs. Bromley."

"You stole my papers. I want to check your bag. You are a thief."

"I didn't touch your papers. I don't even know what papers you're talking about. Is it the newspaper articles? Maybe they are inside the trunk."

"You don't have to pretend with me. You are malicious and evil." She slumped into a rocking chair. "I won't move from here until I find my papers! Where's your purse? I want to inspect your purse!"

To my relief, Molly arrived just then.

"What's going on? Why all the shouting?" she asked, entering the room.

Mrs. Bromley jumped to her feet and pointed a finger at me. "This person stole my papers. Do something about it. Call the police immediately."

"Do you mean your weekly magazines?" Molly asked.

"Yes. We have a thief in the house. Help me search the room and her purse."

Molly held Mrs. Bromley's hand and said softly, "You hid them under the cushion yesterday. Remember? Come with me. I bet they're still there."

"My darling angel. What would I do without you?"

She called Molly a darling angel and called me a thief. I felt humiliated. I watched Molly escort Mrs. Bromley out of the room and I felt very confused. I needed the money and I wanted to work, but not for this unstable, deranged woman. Even though Mrs. Bromley's cruelty was due to illness, it angered me. I always thought I could handle irrational behavior, but Mrs. Bromley's instability proved me wrong. The saying "What goes around comes around" didn't apply to my present situation. When I was well off, I had sympathized with and showed consideration for less-fortunate people. Now that I needed to work, this woman treated me like her doormat. Once, my husband took away my dignity and I fought to regain it; now, Mrs. Bromley was doing a good job of making me feel inferior again.

When Molly returned to the room alone, I asked, "Where's Mrs. Bromley?"

Molly sat next to me on the bed. "She'll be busy for a while reading her beloved tabloids, so now we can talk. What happened?"

I briefed her about Mrs. Bromley's late-night trip into my room with the flashlights and this morning's incident. "I never expected it to be like this. I can't deal with this roller coaster of madness. Her vicious tongue crushes my good intentions." I made a successful effort to hold back the tears.

"To be honest, Lolita, I blame myself for this one. I should have told you about her fixation with those magazines. I assure you that she's not violent." She hesitated and chuckled. "That is, unless she's provoked."

"Well, I certainly didn't provoke her. Now I have to be on the lookout, not knowing when or from where the next surprise will come. I'm sure that in the daytime it is easier and…"

"Oh, no, no!" Molly interrupted. "I also have a lot of problems with her."

"Well, then maybe there's a possibility that we could trade shifts?" I tried, just in case there was a chance.

"I'm awfully sorry, Lolita, but I have a husband, and he wants me home at night. Try to understand that her behavior is due to Alzheimer's, and give her a chance. You'll learn to cope with it."

"I'm usually very patient, but I just lose it with her. I don't think that her main problem is Alzheimer's, I think it's her soul that is sick. She's offensive and mean," I said.

"But Lolita, she's really sick. Also think that she's not used to you yet."

"Still, it's hard to ignore the hatred in her eyes when she looks at me. Yes, I must talk to Mr. Williams."

3

Size and Texture

Full of misgivings, I went to see Mr. Williams to unburden my mind.

"I feel badly that you went through all that, Ms. Rimblas. My grandmother uses the flashlights as entertainment. She waits until it gets dark to play hide and seek with Bowdie around the house." He paused. "She's very theatrical, and sometimes she thinks she's still on the stage. I'm sorry. We should have warned you."

"Yes, it would have helped," I said smiling. "Imagine how I felt on my first night in a strange place to be awakened abruptly by someone standing over me with a blinding light in my face."

"Again, please, accept my apologies. I'll talk to my grandmother before you come back tonight."

I appreciated his good intentions, but I didn't have much hope that things would get any better.

That night, Mrs. Bromley's incessant chatter and repetition made watching television impossible. As my frustration escalated and my patience waned, I reminded myself that it was my job. I was working and being paid for it. Besides, nothing was perfect. After all, it was her right to talk as much s she wanted.

Suddenly, she shut off the television and said, "Tomorrow I'll show you more clippings from my scrapbook."

"God willing, I'd like that." I said, carefully enunciating every word.

"What did you say?"

"I said I'd like that very much."

"Before that."

"God willing?"

"That's a dumb thing to say."

"Why is that dumb?"

"God is always willing." She pointed a finger at me. "You must work for what you want and leave God alone to work on worthwhile affairs. Lazy people think that by asking God, they'll obtain miracles."

I smiled to myself, she made sense. But I wondered why she made such a big deal out of this. Even though her words sounded harsh, she didn't seem angry.

"Do you remember Maurice Chevalier?" she asked.

"Oh, yes. I'm still a big fan of his, and I watch *The Merry Widow* every chance I get."

"Good. Then let me tell you this. We had an affair, and he asked me to marry him, but I refused." She looked at me with a naughty grin and added, "Maurice sent flowers to my dressing room every night."

"How romantic. Why didn't you marry him?"

"He plummeted me into boredom. He knew nothing about the intricacies of passion and romance."

"But he sent you flowers every night. Wasn't that romantic?"

"He was not intense. Flowers without passion are meaningless."

"Did you enjoy his kissing?"

"In a way…but my heart didn't skip a beat."

"I imagined he would send women to heaven."

"He sent me to hell."

I laughed. I enjoyed her British accent and the fine vocabulary she used most of the time. Her romance with Maurice Chevalier was the one thing I didn't mind hearing as many times as she would repeat it.

The next morning, I leaned over Mrs. Bromley to apply her daily glaucoma drop in one eye. The drop landed on her cheek.

"You stupid woman!" she shouted, snatching the bottle from my hand. "Give me the bloody dropper! I can do it better myself. And to think I'm paying good money for this lousy service."

I was taken aback by her sudden outburst and felt my blood boil. I wanted to tell her how nasty she was, and tell her where she could shove her dropper. Her insults hurt so much; still, I couldn't bring myself to say anything. I wanted to cry, to leave this coldhearted woman forever, to quit, but I remembered my situation. A torrent of contradictory feelings consumed me. I wondered where I would find the strength to look at Mrs. Bromley again. Her distorted expression was ingrained in my mind more than her words. I prayed that with time, I would learn not to take her insults to heart. It was going to be difficult, but not impossible.

When I returned that evening, I decided to ignore her. After dinner, I went to my bedroom. Honoring her request, I kept my door open. She appeared several times and glanced around the room.

"Hello, dear, I just want to wish you a good night's sleep."

I felt that indifference in some instances might be what she needed, so I pretended I didn't hear her. She left the room without uttering another word. Bowdie behind her.

It was still dark when I awoke the next morning to hear Mrs. Bromley talking outside my door. "Bowdie," she was saying, "my treasure! Here you are, alone, as if you were an orphan. Has that woman taken you out? No? We both know how selfish she is, but so help me God, she'll pay for neglecting you. I swear."

Could she be talking about me? I jumped out of bed and rushed to the door. In spite of the warm Florida weather, Mrs. Bromley was wearing a heavy winter coat, a hat, gardening gloves, rubber boots and holding a flashlight.

She looked like she was dressed for a blizzard. How sad it was to witness such detachment from reality. God only knew where she was heading, so I grabbed a robe and went after her.

"Good morning, Mrs. Bromley," I called. "Where are you off to so early?"

"Since you don't care about my baby, I'm taking her out."

Was the dog also my responsibility? I was here to take care of her, not that stupid dog. I certainly wasn't going to walk Bowdie at five in the morning.

"Do you know that Bowdie is more regular than me?" she went on, with a better disposition. "And so clever. She goes outside to do her big job. There's never a mess in the house. I'm very proud of her!"

I watched as she stepped outside into a heavy fog, where I couldn't see her, but I did see the beam from the flashlight bobbing up and down. After a few moments, she came back into the house, holding a balled-up paper towel.

"Look at this," she said, unwrapping the towel. "Perfect! Not too soft, not too hard—like two perfect cigars." She walked over to the front door and placed it on the windowsill. "Do not remove this until Molly inspects it."

I was appalled to see how much my life had changed. It was hard to believe that I had once belonged to an elite society. Now I had to examine a dog's feces for a living. It sure was a gigantic leap from the spoiled life I used to live.

She was actually proud of her dog's waste. I couldn't help but reminisce about the time when my children were babies and I had to use rubber gloves and a mask to change their dirty diapers whenever the nanny was off, and now this woman almost rubbed her dog's feces in my face.

Later I asked Molly to explain Mrs. Bromley behavior.

"She has a thing about the size, color, and texture of her dog's doodoo," Molly informed. "Every time I take the little mutt to the park, she demands that I tell her what it looked like. I play along to make her happy. Then I pretend to be excited when I inspect the damn crap she leaves on the windowsill."

"And am I supposed to deal with this?" I asked.

"If you want her to like you, you had better make that dog the center of your attention."

We both laughed about the ridiculous situation we were in.

"Molly, it's funny the way things have turned out for me. I seldom pet any animal. I didn't even allow my children's collie inside the house, and now my job depends on a stupid dog. How ironic," I said thoughtfully. "God's got to be making me pay back for taking for granted what I once had."

"I don't like you women talking in my house." Mrs. Bromley's shrill voice interrupted us. "You are both conspiring against me. Molly, you leave now, and the other Molly may stay," she demanded.

How amusing her confusion turned out to be. I left not knowing if I were Molly or Lolita.

The second I arrived that evening, Mrs. Bromley handed me the dog on its leash.

"You take Baby for a walk in the park. And this is for her big job." She gave me a plastic bag and a napkin.

"Where's the park?"

"Four houses down that way. Hurry up and go. It's getting dark."

When I came back fifteen minutes later, she was waiting by the door.

"Well, how was it?" she asked.

I tried to be evasive. There was no way I was going to describe her dog's droppings.

"We had a very nice walk."

"What do you mean 'a nice walk'? How was my baby's big job?"

"Oh, fine," I said, trying not to laugh.

"How big?" She held out a finger. "This big? Bigger? Skinny? Was it fat?"

Feeling ridiculous, I pointed at my wrist and cried out, "This big!" But I really wanted to give her the finger.

"How many trophies? One or two…?"

"Two," I said, holding up two fingers for victory.

She clapped her hands. "Fantastic! Where are they?"

"I threw them away."

"You did what! Where is your brain? Why do you think I gave you a plastic bag?"

"I'm sorry. I didn't know."

"The rule is that every time Bowdie does her business, you bring it to me. This time, I'll let it go, but I must say, you have no initiative at all. Baby," she said, hugging the dog, "you are a genius! Now it's Mommy's toddy time. Come on, Molly."

"Will you please try to remember? My name is Lolita," I said for the hundredth time.

"Will you please—your majesty Lo-li-ta—hurry up with my drinky-poo? Have one yourself, and who knows? You might get rid of your sour face."

After our drinks, the alcohol relaxed her, which had the same effect on me. But all that lasted until food killed it.

At nine, I went to her bedroom. She was sitting in front of a mirror, flossing her teeth, her gray hair cascading down her shoulders.

"I came to say good night," I said, standing at the door.

"What did you say?" she shouted.

"I said, I came to say good night," I repeated.

"Now, what did you say?" she shouted louder.

"Nothing!" I thought she couldn't hear me, so I shouted back just as loud. "I'll see you tomorrow."

"You don't have to shout," she said, continuing to floss. "You said you wanted to say good night."

I bristled. "Mrs. Bromley, I think you just like to play games."

"What did you say?"

"Good night," I said, and walked away.

Half an hour later, while I was in bed watching TV, she showed up at my door.

"Good night. God bless."

"God bless you too," I said.

She came closer. "Did you say something?"

"God bless you!" I repeated.

"Bravo! That's what I thought."

I was relishing my solitude, thinking she was already in bed for the evening, but she reappeared at my door four more times, saying, "I came to say *re-good night.*"

As she stood in the doorway, wearing a transparent negligee, I thought she looked incredible for a woman her age…actually, for any age. She still had a sculpted figure, not unlike her statue in the living room.

At about four in the morning, I was headed for the bathroom when I heard a strange high-pitched noise. I tried to figure out where it was coming from and what it was, but all of a sudden, the noise stopped. It didn't sound like an alarm clock or anything familiar. I continued toward the bathroom, when the noise started again. This time it sounded like it was coming from Mrs. Bromley's room. I started in her direction, but by the time I got there, it had stopped. As soon as I got back to my bedroom, the noise started again. I hurried back to her room, which was faintly illuminated by a night-light. I looked over to the night table and realized the noise was coming from her hearing aid. I tiptoed across the room and was just about to pick up the hearing aid when Mrs. Bromley woke up and screamed, "Who's there?"

"It's me," I answered.

She grabbed her flashlight and pointed it at my face. "Get away from me!"

I froze.

"It's you!" she shouted. "Well, you won't get my jewelry! Go away, thief!"

I switched on the overhead light. "I came in to shut off your hearing aid." I showed it to her, but she snatched it away from me. I expected her to hit me, and flinched.

"Get out of my room, thief!" she continued to scream. "I'll tell my grandson, you can be sure of that! We have a bloody thief in the house!"

"I only wanted to turn off your hearing aid, it was squealing." I tried to explain.

"I don't know what you are saying. Get out!"

"That's because you don't have your hearing aids in!" I screamed, and stormed out of the room.

Was it possible that I was going to live through a nightmare like this every night? I counted sheep. I prayed. I went to the kitchen for hot milk. Nothing helped.

The first light of morning found me wide-awake with my heart pounding. My head throbbed and my neck was getting stiffer by the second. I just wanted to get out of this house. I didn't foresee things getting better. It was one thing to have to deal with a forgetful, complex person, and an entirely different thing to have to deal with a crazy, paranoid one. I decided to quit. Now that I had gained some experience, it would be easier to find a job taking care of a normal person. I got out of bed with a pounding headache. Reluctantly, I prepared her breakfast and took it to her room. Her face brightened when she saw me.

"Darling," she said, and clapped her hands. "How nice of you to bring my breakfast. Did you sleep well?"

I wanted to shout, *No! How could I?* Instead I said, "Yes, I did. Thank you kindly."

"What did you say?"

"I said yes thank you," I shouted.

To think that I worried so much all night and had been hurt because she called me a "thief." Now she didn't even remember. *God, please, keep reminding me that she's sick when she insults me and, furthermore, remind me to turn the other cheek and to keep a stiff upper lip.*

4

Church

Mrs. Bromley and I were having our evening drink when the doorbell rang.

"Don't open it," she said when I started for the door. "I don't receive callers on Thursdays."

"But today is Monday," I said.

"You don't know anything, not even what day it is."

The doorbell continued to ring.

"May I see who it is, Mrs. Bromley? It could be your grandson."

"Gary has a key. I don't want to see anyone today. Bowdie, stop that barking!"

"Good evening, Betty," a tall woman said as she walked over to Mrs. Bromley and kissed her on both cheeks.

"How did you get in?" Mrs. Bromley asked coldly.

"Darling, I have a key. Remember?"

"Gary is the only one with a key to my house. What are you doing here?"

"I'm visiting my grandson, and I came to say hello."

"Okay, you said hello; now say good-bye and get out. And don't dare to bring that brat over here. He touches everything with his dirty hands."

The woman, a middle-aged blonde, backed away. "So you're in one of those bad moods again," she said, with a straight face.

"And you made it worse."

"I had a bad day myself, Betty." She sighed and looked at me. "I'm Jane, Mr. Williams' mother, and you must be Lolita. I'm very glad to meet you."

"I'm glad to meet you too," I said.

"It makes me sick when she acts like that. Sorry we had to meet under these circumstances."

"Molly!" Mrs. Bromley shouted. "Would you please tell that person to get out of my house?"

I felt embarrassed. It wasn't my place to tell Mrs. Williams to leave.

Jane rolled her eyes and started for the door. "You have my sympathy, Lolita. You certainly have your job cut out for you."

Mrs. Bromley said, "Stop talking, and Molly, make sure she doesn't steal anything."

Jane winked at me as she walked out. I regretted the way Mrs. Bromley had behaved, but at the same time I was selfishly relieved to see that I wasn't the only one she mistreated.

"It wasn't polite of you to treat Mrs. Williams like that," I said, sitting across from her.

"That is none of your business."

"If you want your family to visit you, you'd better change your attitude and be nice to them."

"Keep your opinion to yourself until I ask for it," she snapped. "That is, *if* I ever ask for it—which I never will."

She leaned over and raised the volume on the TV. For once, I didn't care if it was too loud because at least she was quiet and it gave me the welcome opportunity to spend time by myself.

That night, I kept thinking about Mrs. Bromley's daughter-in-law, Jane. I couldn't make up my mind whether I liked her or not. Though our meeting had been brief, there was something about her that intimidated me. Certainly she had a strong personality.

I had always believed that people were not given more than they could handle in life. If God had sent me this cross, it was because He knew I was capable of carrying it. When I was married to Mauricio, who was unpredictable and unreasonable, I had gotten through stressful times by using common sense. I hoped that those experiences would help me cope with Mrs. Bromley.

Due to illness or not, she kept me on edge.

I wanted to gain insight into what made her disagreeable and to do my best to understand all I could about Alzheimer's. I also wanted to be more tolerant of her fluctuating moods. I prayed for the endurance to climb the mountain, no matter how steep. With my husband, it had taken fifteen years, but I knew Mrs. Bromley and I didn't have that long.

I wished I had more communication with Mr. Williams and his wife; there were many things I would like to know about Mrs. Bromley before Alzheimer's struck her. I tried to converse with Molly, but Mrs. Bromley insisted that I leave as soon as Molly arrived. In order for us to talk, Molly and I agreed to meet at Howard Park, where she took the dog upon her arrival every morning.

I needed to let off steam, so I went to the park and waited for Molly there. As soon as she arrived with Bowdie, I welcomed her and got right to the point.

"That woman is driving me crazy. She talks incessantly, and repeats every-thing." I spoke fast; afraid I wouldn't have enough time to unburden myself. "She has the television on all night, so I hardly get any sleep. In fact, when I get up in the morning the darn thing is still blasting."

Molly laughed. "Try to ignore her constant yakking and the blasting TV, then maybe you'd be able to enjoy her when she's in a good mood, which is apparently in the early morning. By the way, why don't you try earplugs?"

"I tried, but the noise goes right through them."

"Tell her you won't sit with her unless she turns down the TV."

"I did. She turns it down and then turns it up even louder."

Molly shook her head. "Well, if I were you, I'd go to your room and close the door."

"I can't. She orders me to keep it open."

"Lolita, I give up. I'm out of suggestions, and you have one big problem."

"If it were only one! There are so many." I pushed back my hair and went on, "Did I tell you that she pops into my room constantly when I'm trying to sleep? If she sees I'm on the phone, she tells me to stop babbling and asks if it's long dis-tance. My sister-in-law was so right when she warned me about this job. She said that nobody gives money away. One way or another, you work hard for every dime."

"How right she was," Molly said. "Mr. Williams pays well, but the truth is that putting up with his grandmother doesn't have a price." Molly sat forward on the bench as she watched how Bowdie sniffed the grass. "How about making your phone calls after she's asleep?"

"I never know when she's sleeping. Even if her light is off and she's in bed, she gets up and comes in my room. By the time she falls asleep, I'm drained and don't want to talk to anyone. Besides that, it would be too late to make a call."

"Yeah. I forgot. That's why they couldn't retain help for the night shift. I guess she is better during the day, but like some other illnesses, she gets worse at night. They call it 'sun downing.'"

"I thought it was going to be the other way around," I said, "that we would both sleep at night. But wait, I haven't told you everything yet. She sets the ther-mostat at eighty-two and I can hardly stand the heat. I turn it down, and she turns it up, so I have to sleep with the windows open, but even that doesn't help because there's no breeze."

"It sounds to me like you're fed up. Please don't tell me you're quitting."

"No, don't worry. I guess I'm just venting. I hate to bother Mr. Williams with my complaints again. I suppose I just need time to adjust to the situation and come up with my own solution."

"I'm sorry, Lolita."

"Oh, Molly, forgive me for bothering you."

"It's okay. I know you need a sounding board." She paused for a moment. "But you know, I think you should talk to Mr. Williams before you explode." She thought for a moment. "Now, forget Mrs. Bromley, and let's talk about you. I know you're divorced and have never worked before, but that's about all I know about you. What do you do for fun?" she asked, grinning.

"I belong to Jane Olson's singles travel club, and we have parties in different houses at least once a month. We have gourmet dinners from different countries. I offer my house once in a while for the parties, and we hire entertainers. I go every Saturday to Pinawor, a writers' group. I wrote two screenplays, and I self-published a book called *Maite*."

"Wonderful! What is *Maite* about?"

"*Maite* is the nickname for Maria Teresa. Although the novel is fiction, it's based in great part on my own experiences in Mexico. It's about power and corruption and the impossible love between people of two different social classes. It takes place in Mexico City, Acapulco, and Puerto Vallarta. People who have read it said that they couldn't put it down."

"Good for you. Are you writing anything now?"

"I'm working on another book: *One Step from Freedom*. It's about my life in Cuba and how I got to the United States."

"How interesting! I'd love to read some of your work."

"I'll give you a copy of *Maite* and some pages of what I'm writing now."

"Whoa, Lolita, you certainly have an interesting life. So you are Cuban. How did you get to the United States?"

"I married a Spanish Jew and we lived in Spain for two years, then we settled in Mexico. After many years of living under his yoke, I rebelled and wanted to live a more meaningful life. He almost killed me, and I was forced to leave my home and kids."

"Oh, Lolita, that's awful. What did you do?"

"First, I went to a friend's house. My friend helped me go to New York, where an attorney handled our divorce and I received a nice settlement. I put in a good down payment for a house in Florida and he agreed in a generous alimony. I fought for my kids, but Mauricio threatened to take them abroad and away from me forever. Mexico is corrupt, and money weighs more than justice…" I began to cry and couldn't go on.

I felt Molly's arms on my shoulders. "Lolita, I only wanted you to feel better, and I made things worse. Come on; take your mind off the past. I'll tell you a little about me, how about it?"

I interrupted, "I want you to know that I have a great relationship with my kids," I said, wiping off my tears. "They are all grown up now; this was a long time ago, but it still hurts. We call each other on the phone daily." I forced a smile. "Now tell me about you."

"It's very boring but not tragic. I'm happily married and I have two adorable kids." She jumped to her feet. "Lolita, I didn't realize it's getting late, and I have to clean up after Bowdie. We'll continue this conversation another day. I'll see you tomorrow."

As soon as I arrived home, I called Mr. Williams.

"I understand, Lolita," he said when I told him my complaints.

"Alzheimer's is only part of the problem; her strong will and superiority complex make it worse. I'll do whatever it takes to keep her away from a nursing home as long as I can. Now, what can we do to make things better?"

"Oh, Lord, it's hard to say. I worry so much—there are so many problems. The worse one is that I can't sleep, it's so hot—"

"Look, let's try this," he interrupted gently. "I'll ask the doctor if we can increase her sleeping pill dosage; that way, both of you will get more sleep. Also, I'm going to post rules all over the house to help her remember." He paused. "Something else, Lolita: you don't have to call me to solve these problems anymore. From now on, you're on your own. You have our blessings and trust, so don't let my grandmother push you around. Don't hesitate to show her you're in control."

I was speechless. I needed to digest the meaning of his words. Me alone bearing the responsibility for Mrs. Bronley? Me in charge?

"Do you need time to think about this?" he asked.

"I appreciate your trust," I finally said, "but I'm not sure I can do it without your help."

"Don't underestimate yourself. I'm sure you have the capacity and the guts to deal with my grandmother. I have faith in you."

I sighed. "That's quite a responsibility, Mr. Williams."

"You can do it. Call me Gary, please," he said emphatically.

"I'll try, Mr. Williams—I mean, Gary. I'll do my best,"

I knew that I had to find a way to control Mrs. Bromley, and I knew it would be hard work but I must try. I imagined him smiling when he said, "You'll do an excellent job taming my incorrigible grandmother."

I hung up the phone very concerned. He had used the word "taming." It was strange that in such a short time, he trusted me enough to place his grandmother in my care and without his supervision. *At least*, I thought, *he could have suggested a method for me to follow.* How would I make her do what I want? Since I hated arguments, I usually backed away from them. If I were going to "tame" Mrs. Bromley, as he said, I would need to stand up to her. I anticipated a future with enough conflict to last me a lifetime.

After thinking it over, I realized what this would mean in regards to her usual threat: "My grandson will hear about this, and he'll get rid of you, then I won't have to see your face anymore." Now I wouldn't have to worry about losing my job anymore. I'll be free to be more assertive with Mrs. Bromley, and able to use my own common sense. Who knows? Maybe she would react positively to that.

I was about to pour myself a glass of water when Mrs. Bromley called, "Molly, come see what Gary did."

"Do you think that one day you're going to remember that my name is Lolita?" I snapped and immediately regretted it. I hurried into the living room.

"It's up to you to remember your name. Come with me." She pointed to the note that Mr. Williams had written and posted on her bedroom door and began to read it. "Do not go to Lolita's room after nine o'clock. Keep the TV low. Don't interrupt phone conversations. Keep the thermostat at seventy-eight."

She glared at me. "There are bloody notes like this all over the house. There's even one stuck to the TV. I think Gary's head isn't working right these days. I'm going to leave them where they are, only to make him happy."

After that, things changed a little. Now she only came into my room to ask for help finding her clock, her eyeglasses, her hairnet, the appointment book, and even the dog. As for the heat, I kept lowering the temperature, and she kept raising it. The TV volume went up and went down. There was no change with the telephone, since she was obsessed with what she thought were long-distance calls.

Two days later I was about to get into bed when Mrs. Bromley entered my room.

"Look, Molly," she said, sticking out her tongue. "This is what I'm going to do with these ridiculous notes that someone wrote." She shredded the papers into tiny bits and threw them in the air. "And this is for you, Molly." She held the bottom of her nightgown, hummed "The Blue Danube," and danced around the room like a child.

My heart went out to Mrs. Bromley as I watched her dancing with Alzheimer's.

The next morning, as I was getting ready to leave, Molly arrived and declared, "Lolita, I'm sorry to tell you this on such short notice, but something important turned up and I need to take tomorrow off. Could you please work for me? Oh…Mrs. Bromley is calling. I'll meet you at the park and tell you more about it."

"Good! I'll see you there."

I left for the park to wait for Molly, thinking that I was happy to have the extra pay, but not happy to have an extra day with Mrs. Bromley. When Molly arrived with Bowdie, I told her I gladly accepted but with only one condition.

"I go to mass on Sundays," I explained. "Do you think Mrs. Bromley will be okay while I'm gone? I'll go to the seven o'clock mass and I'll be back in less than an hour."

"Sure, I think she'll be okay. Just leave a note and tell her what time you'll be back."

"Does Mr. Williams know I'll be working tomorrow?"

"Oh, yeah, no problem. He doesn't mind."

Sunday morning, before I left for church, I checked on Mrs. Bromley. At first, I thought she was sleeping, but when she opened her eyes, I asked if she would like to go to church with me.

"What?" she shouted.

I handed her the hearing aids. "Will you please put on your hearing aids? I need to talk to you." I used my hands in order to help her understand what I wanted.

"Do you want to go to church with me?"

"What kind of church?" she asked. "I mean what denomination?"

"Catholic," I answered.

"No, I'm not interested. I'm Anglican."

I tried to coax her. "Come with me, Mrs. Bromley. They're similar. I'm sure you'll like it."

"That kind of service doesn't amuse me."

"But you don't go to church to be amused. You go to pray to God."

She sat up and shouted, "I'm free to go to church for any reason I damn well bloody choose, so don't interfere in my life! I don't like Catholic preachers, and I don't like Catholics either."

"Well, I'm sure that they would like you."

"I'm sure that they wouldn't, and I'm not discussing it with you. In fact, it's none of your business. Is that clear?"

"Yes. It's clear," I said, thinking she had a point. "So if you don't mind, I'll be going now."

"You're going whether I mind it or not, so go on, go ahead! Get out of here! The sooner, the better."

"I'll be back in a few minutes. Please wait for me in bed until I come back."

"What did you say?"

"Never mind." I wrote a note and placed it in her hand along with her glasses.

She read it aloud. "Dear Mrs. Bromley, I'm going to church, but I'll be back shortly. Wait for me in bed until I get back. God bless you. Love, Lolita."

She asked, "Who's Lolita?"

I shook my head and said, "I'm Lolita. Do you understand my note? Will you please stay put until I come back?"

"I'm not an idiot," she said, crumbling the note.

I wrote another one and stuck it to the refrigerator. I left feeling uneasy about her being alone. On the other hand, I needed to go to church and it wouldn't take long. I rationalized that there was nothing wrong about leaving her for something as important as fulfilling God's commandment. My husband hadn't allowed me to go to church, and now I felt indebted to God. I wanted to make up for it by worshiping God in church, at least every Sunday.

I couldn't concentrate during mass, so I decided to leave early.

When I got back to the house, I was shocked to find it empty. My heart sank. Where on earth could she be? *O God, what have I done? How could I have left a senile, old lady alone, while under my care?* It was the same as leaving a baby unattended.

A chill went through me. After I searched the house, I drove around the neighborhood while my panic escalated. I felt so guilty. If anything happened to her, I would die!

Mrs. Bromley was nowhere to be found. I realized that I had to tell Mr. Williams what happened so he could call the police and report her missing. I was terrified of what he would say.

I visualized the police searching for the poor old lady, and I could almost hear the wailing sirens. I envisioned Mrs. Bromley's body lying on the side of the road and me on cuffs in a jail cell somewhere.

If only I could wake up from this nightmare!

I pulled up to Mr. Williams's driveway and hurried to the front door but hesitated before ringing the bell. What would I say? What if I forgot to speak English, which sometimes happened when I was nervous? I finally mustered up enough courage and was about to ring the bell when the door opened. I felt the urge to run, but Mr. Williams's friendly smile stopped me.

"I don't know how to tell you," I stammered. "I am so—

"Don't worry, Lolita. My grandmother's here."

I took a deep breath and said, "Oh, thank God. I'm so sorry. I'm so embarrassed."

"It's okay. Come inside." I followed him to the living room. "Have a seat," he said, pointing to the couch.

My knees were shaking and I was grateful to sit down. He sat across from me and asked, "What happened?"

On the verge of tears, I tried to explain, "I went to church…" I cleared my throat. "I told her not to get out of bed. I left her a note. Oh, Mr. Williams, it won't happen again."

He started to laugh. "She came over and was banging on the door, still in her nightgown, demanding to know who had left her the note. She was looking for Molly. I couldn't figure out what was going on. I knew that Molly was off and that you were taking care of her."

"Oh, Mr. Williams, now I know what happened. I signed the note 'Lolita,' but she calls me Molly. She never remembers my name."

"That explains it, and now you realize that she can't be left alone anymore." He winked when he said, "Well, Molly, do you agree?"

"Yes, Mr. Williams, Molly agrees, Lopeta and Lolita also agree." I felt relieved that things hadn't gone any further. Hopefully I had learned my lesson. "Now, would you like me to take her home?"

"No. Why don't you take the rest of the day off? Right now, she doesn't want to see you ever again. But tonight, she'll be happy to see you."

I asked myself if I ever would be able to control her as Molly could. Would I be able to tame her like Mr. Williams had said?

Only time would tell.

5

Alzheimer's in a Nutshell

I still felt guilty about leaving Mrs. Bromley alone. Even if Mr. Williams had ended up laughing, I was so upset that I didn't feel like going right home. Although he was very understanding, I wondered if he would trust me again. Even worse, I was afraid that he might change his mind and fire me. I decided to relax at the beach and ignore my nagging thoughts. Lying down on the sand with the sun on my face, I was lulled by the sound of the receding waves. They slowly washed away my sense of guilt.

On my way to work that evening, my spirits were high. I was happy to be alive and grateful to be healthy. I had a new sense of purpose and was proud to have a paying job. I was determined not to take anything for granted anymore.

It filled me with joy to see houses lit up everywhere, announcing that Christmas was just around the corner. Brightly decorated homes and businesses gave me the impression they were competing with each other. A winter flock of snow-birds [the human kind] brought bumper-to-bumper traffic. As I struggled my way through, I thought of Emerson's philosophy that one must give up some things in order to gain others. My trade-off was to work for a demanding, spoiled woman, who needed me as much as I needed her, for the benefit of financial independence and a sense of pride and purpose.

Up until now my ex-husband had been the most difficult person I ever had to deal with. Over years of patience and understanding, I had learned to cope with his challenging personality. Now my closeness to Mrs. Bromley gave me the opportunity to draw from those experiences. I knew it would take time, but if it was true that love conquered all, I was ready to shower Mrs. Bromley with love to prove it.

When I arrived at the house, she opened the door and I was surprised to find myself hugging her, only to feel her body stiffen like a brick wall. I almost kissed her, but she pushed me away and walked into the living room. I don't know what got into me, I should have known better. Maybe the reason I wanted to kiss her was the panic I felt this morning at the thought of losing her.

"Go away," she grumbled. "I've had enough! I've had enough!"

"What's wrong, Mrs. Bromley?" I asked timidly, thinking she was referring to the church incident.

"If they think they can do this to me, they don't know me. I will not take this anymore! I'll move back to my old house. I have no one here." She spun around and shook a finger at me. "And you're no better. You left me alone all afternoon. I don't even know why you are here."

"I'm here to take care of you," I said.

"It's too late now. I was alone all day."

"But, I thought you were with your grandson."

"Don't you understand English?" she shouted as she paced back and forth. "I'm telling you I was left alone all day! Do you understand what I am saying? If it wasn't for faithful Bowdie, I'd be dead. You would have found a decomposing body."

"But thank God, you're not dead," I was quick to add.

"No thanks to you, and you probably would have been happy if I were dead. Then you could have the whole house for yourself."

"You're wrong. I'd be very upset if anything happened to you, Mrs. Bromley."

"But I could have been kidnapped."

Yes, I thought, *and after one night with you, they would have returned you in the morning.* I smiled to myself. *And on top of it, they'd pay me to get rid of you.*

"But," I said, "you weren't kidnapped, and you weren't hurt. Now I'm here and I'll stay with you as long as you need me, so don't worry anymore, I won't leave you alone."

"Really? Will you really stay here?" she asked, almost like a child. "Will you, really? Yes? Do you promise?"

"Yes, Mrs. Bromley, I promise."

"Say it again."

"I won't leave you."

"Oh, yes, Molly, don't leave me. I hate being alone. I really missed you."

"Not a word about it anymore. I'll be with you all night." I could see how frightened she was, and I felt my heart fill with compassion.

She motioned for me to sit on the sofa, and I did.

She stopped pacing and sat beside me. "Do you know why I don't want to be alone?" She clutched at her chest. "I dread being by myself in case of a heart attack. I've suffered enough because Gary screwed me out of my fortune, and now I have to depend on him. What's worse, it's like I should be grateful because he gives me the gift of my own money. Do you think that's fair?"

I didn't want to be involved in a family dispute, so I smiled reassuringly and shrugged.

Suddenly, she got up and started pacing again. "He bought this house with my money and without my consent. I hate this bloody house. I want to go back to France. My friends are there, and I was happy with them. Tell me, whose side are you on?"

I wondered if she was telling the truth. Was it another one of her delusions? It bothered me that I didn't know more about her and about this awful disease. I decided to call my son-in-law in Minnesota that night. As a neurologist, he'd be able to shed some light on this illness.

"Molly, I'm waiting!" she shouted. "Are you with them or with me? Speak up! On what side of the fence are you?"

I wanted to change the subject, so I said, "Did you enjoy your visit with your great-grandson? What's his name?"

"Oh, Lord! Am I speaking Chinese? They left me all alone! They are mean to me. I want to know whose side you are on."

"Look, Mrs. Bromley, I care for you very much, but I don't know anything about your family and this particular situation. It wouldn't be fair for me to have an opinion."

She glared at me. Her face was filled with hatred. "My son and my grandson ripped me off."

"Mr. Williams told me to make your happiness my first priority," I said quickly. "He wants you to be happy."

"Are you naive or stupid?" she shouted. "Can't you tell when people are sincere? They're acting. But of course, you don't know them." She leaned closer to me and whispered, "They come at night and take whatever they want. Last night, my grandson took the pillows from under my head while I was sleeping to give them to his guest."

What she said was so ridiculous that it made me feel sad. I was totally at a loss for words. I looked at her with compassion, wishing I could hold her tight and brush away her fears. She needed love, and I had a lot to give; maybe one day she would accept it. I leaned a little closer to her and placed my hand over hers squeezing gently, then removed it quickly, not giving her time to pull away.

"Mrs. Bromley, your grandson seems sincere. He's the kind of person who looks into your eyes when he speaks. To me, that means you can trust him."

"If you don't know what you are talking about, keep your mouth shut."

Ignoring her request, I went on. "He says it doesn't matter how much it costs, he wants to give you the best care. He asks me every day how you're doing." Although it wasn't exactly true, I hoped it would appease her. Mr. Williams never asked for a daily report, but I didn't mind exaggerating if it brought her some peace. "I don't think there's enough money in the world to pay for someone's love and care and your grandson loves you very much."

"So you really believe him? How gullible you are. He puts up with me because the money he's spending is mine. Of course it's easy for him to be generous with my money."

"Still, he's spending it on you. He is investing your money wisely. He's young. He could be using your money for gambling, drinking, or chasing women. Instead, he works overtime to make your money grow."

"My money grow? My bloody foot! You know, they are always telling secrets behind my back. Everybody whispers so I can not hear what they are saying. Do you think that it is proper manners? You're wasting my time, so let's move on." She stopped pacing and clapped her hands. "Now it's time for my drinkypoo, and be sure to make it very strong."

I fixed a strong drink for her and a welcome double scotch for myself, expecting a more relaxing evening.

Later that night, I locked myself in the bathroom and placed a collect call to my son-in-law, Rafael. After exchanging pleasantries and inquiring about the family I explained to Rafael what my situation was with Mrs. Bromley.

"Look, Lolita," he said. "I'm not an expert on Alzheimer's, but I'll tell you a little bit of what I do know. First, it's a progressive disease of the brain. It is one type of dementia that causes deterioration of intellectual faculties, like memory, concentration, and judgment. These cause emotional disturbances and personality changes."

"Alzheimer's and dementia are the same thing?" I asked

"Well, yes and no; there are many causes of dementia, and Alzheimer's is the most common cause. The diagnosis can only definitively be made on autopsy. Grossly, there is cerebral atrophy, including hippocampal atrophy, and ventricular enlargement. Pathologically there are neuritic senile plaques, neurofibrillary tangles, and amyloid deposition. In the early stages, short-term memory is the first to go and the ability to perform routine tasks is also affected. But unless you can examine the brain it is hard to know if a patient is suffering from dementia of the Alzheimer's type or from some other type of dementia."

"Excuse me Rafael," I interrupted, "in case you've forgotten, I' haven't attended medical school."

"I am sorry, Lolita, I get carried away. Basically, what this means is that, as the disease spreads throughout the brain, it affects judgment, causes emotional out-bursts and language impairment. Towards the end communication is completely lost; the patient is bedridden and totally dependent upon others."

"How terrible." I sighed. "So there is no cure?"

"Unfortunately, there's no cure, but scientists at the Mayo Clinic are starting to detect the onset of dementia at the earliest stages; before reaching the stage of Alzheimer's, they call it Mild Cognitive Impairment (MCI). By detecting this abnormal aging early on, therapeutic interventions can be started earlier, with the hope of slowing the progression of this devastating disease. Actually, some studies show that Non-Steroidal Anti-Inflammatory Drugs and vitamin E may delay the onset of AD in high risk patients. Of course, it probably wouldn't hurt to keep the patient engaged and active, and also eating a balanced, low in cholesterol diet."

"What can we do?" I asked.

"There are a lot of things we can all do to improve our mental capacity and fight dementia. I don't know if it is too late for Mrs. Bromley, but it wouldn't hurt to try. It is crucial to remain emotionally involved. Leisure activities that combine physical, mental and social activity are the most likely to prevent dementia. I know of one study that looked at about one thousand elderly people and those who were more physically and mentally active had a lower risk for developing dementia."

"Really?"

"Yes, and also keep in mind that it is very important to have a lot of loving support, not only for the patient, but for the care-taker too.

"This sounds encouraging, thank you Rafael."

"You are very welcome, Lolita. But also, you should talk to Olivia, because I assume Mrs. Bromley can't hear well either."

"Oh sure! I'd love to talk to *mi morenita linda.*"

Olivia, my oldest daughter, is an audiologist and Rafael's wife. She was in school getting her doctorate degree.

"*Hola mamita linda,*" she said in a crispy voice. "I had been thinking what you told me about Mrs. Bromley's incident with her hearing aids. There isn't a lot I can do from here without seeing her. Do you know if she opens the hearing aid's battery door at night?

"Well, I have no idea, *mi reinita*. Should she open it?" I asked.

"Yes mom, that way you turn the hearing aids off and it won't squeal at night. Also the batteries will last longer."

"Good. I'll make sure she does it."

"Another thing you can do is to check the battery often to make sure it still works. She might be walking around with dead hearing aids."

"How do I do that?" I asked

"Well, you get a battery tester. Also you can cup the hearing aids into your hand and if they squeal the battery is OK. If there is no squealing put in a new battery and see if you get the squeal. Also, if the hearing aids squeal while they're in her ears she might think the hearing aids are "talking to her" and get nervous." For this you need to make sure there isn't wax in her ears. It could also be due to other problems, that's why it's so important to take her regularly to the audiologist.

"Okay, chiquita linda, I'll do that."

"The last thing mamita, and this is very important, you would not believe how closely related dementia and hearing loss are. I have seen so many patients that were unresponsive, depressed and with advanced dementia and cognitive decline, bounce back once they had well fitted hearing aids, people benefit more when used in both ears. So *mamita*, take Mrs. Bromley to her audiologist and make sure she hears well."

"But Olivia, Molly is the one taking her to her doctors' appointments. Remember? I've the night shift."

"Then, just tell Molly everything I told you."

"Of course, I will. Thank you, morenita linda."

"Love you, good night. Oh hold on, Rafael thought of something else, bye."

My ear felt hot so I turned the receiver to the other ear and peeked out the door to make sure Mrs. Bromley wasn't coming. The coast was clear, so confidently I continue with our conversation.

"Yes Rafael, you wanted to add something?"

"Yes Lolita. It just occurred to me that you are a writer and she was a performer, so why not tell her that you want to write a book and you need to know more about her life. You both can play-act stories of her youth when she certainly had happier times. Her present is scary, but her past is safe. Read books out loud; tell her stories. The only good thing about this awful disease is that you don't have to rack your brain thinking of new stories, you can tell her the same over and over. It's a good way to practice your English."

"This all makes a lot of sense," I said gratefully.

"Mrs. Bromley is very lucky to have the money to pay for a private caregiver."

"But Rafael, I'm not a nurse nor a caregiver. I was hired as a companion. I didn't know anything about Alzheimer's when I took this job."

"Call it whatever you want, but you are still a caregiver, whether you want to be or not. She's going to need more love and understanding than physical care. Expect to be her companion and caregiver in a very long journey to nowhere."

"I don't like the sound of that. It gives me the chills."

"Life can be so cruel. Sometimes I wonder why with so much garbage in the world I was given such a small broom to sweep it away. We must all do what we can. That is my advice, *querida* Lolita. Place yourself in her shoes. Understand what awaits her. The woman has a future without any dignity. It's one hellish living death before dying. But the one thing that Alzheimer's can't strip away is your love and friendship.

"Thanks, Rafael. You gave me a lot to think about. I really appreciate your help."

After I hung up, I went to my room and was grateful that Mrs. Bromley wasn't at my door looking for me. Now all I had to do was to stop and remember what Rafael and Olivia said whenever the time came.

First thing tomorrow morning I will tell Molly to take Mrs. Bromley to her audiologist to have her hearing and hearing aids checked. I will also share with her all the interesting and helpful things Rafael and Olivia told me.

6

Quitting

Later that night, Mrs. Bromley came to my room, dressed only in her underwear. I was shocked to see that her head was covered with a pantyhose, and the legs were hanging down on each side. I felt a mixture of humor and sorrow at the bizarre sight.

"Do you like the way my hat looks, or does it look better this way?" She tied the legs into a bow under her chin. I couldn't contain myself any longer and laughed out loud.

"What is so bloody funny?"

"Oh, nothing. You look cute."

"How kind, Molly. Thank you. Would you like to try it on?"

"Oh, no, no," I answered quickly, and pointed to the clock. "It's too late."

"*Bon*, then hurry up," she said nervously. "Be an angel and help me find my torch?'

"Your what?"

"My torch."

"Do you mean a candle?"

"*Mon Dieu*, are you an imbecile? Forget that bloody candle, and let's look for my torch right now."

Not knowing what I was looking for, I followed her to the bedroom and began opening drawers and looking under furniture, searching for whatever a torch was.

"Darling," she said, "I'm going to bed. Whenever you find the torch, bring it to me."

It irritated me that I had to look for her torch while she relaxed in bed, but then I felt guilty for being annoyed. While looking in her closet, I remembered a similar incident that happened many years ago when Mauricio and I had first moved to Mexico and we rented a furnished house. I had asked Lupe, the maid, to bring me a slice of *fruta bomba*. She said, "*Si, señora*," and left. She was taking too long, so I went to the kitchen to see what was keeping her. Every drawer and door in the cabinets had been flung open. Pots and pans were scattered over the counters. When I asked what happened, she said she couldn't find it. Then I asked what she was looking for.

"I don't know," she said. "I'm looking for that thing you wanted me to get you."

She hadn't known what she was looking for, but she had looked, just the same to please me. Now I was doing the same thing to please Mrs. Bromley. Finally I gave up and went over to her bed. "It's two o'clock in the morning," I said, looking at the clock.

"Well, what're you doing here now? Don't ever wake me up this early again."

"Then we'll look for your torch tomorrow."

"What torch?"

"The torch you told me to look for."

"How stupid can you be? I have it here." She burst out laughing, as she held up a flashlight.

I was confused and not amused at all. I thought that I preferred to be called Molly than stupid. "But you asked me for a torch."

"I have my torch," she held out the flashlight. "Don't you know what a torch is?"

"No. I thought that was a flashlight or a lantern."

"Now you know. You may retire now, I want to sleep."

My thoughts went back to Lupe, and I thought I should have explained to her that *fruta bomba* was the name for "papaya" in Havana, Cuba. She must have felt as stupid then as I felt stupid now.

Early the next morning, I heard Mrs. Bromley screaming at the dog. She stood outside my bedroom door, fully dressed.

"Good morning, Mrs. Bromley. How are you?" I asked, wanting to go back to sleep.

"Thanks to you, there's nothing good about this morning." Her eyes narrowed and her lips pulled up. "I'm ashamed," she said. "Now I'll be on the neighbors' blacklist. I do not want my grandson to find out about you. I can't believe this is happening in my exclusive neighborhood."

I was fully awake now and curious. "What did I do?" I asked. "What's wrong?"

"You need to be a decent person or leave my house. You put me to shame. You're a disgrace."

Her barrage of accusations outraged me. I wondered what I could have done to trigger this attack. "But what did I do?" I managed to ask again.

"How dare you leave your car unlocked?"

"What? My car unlocked?" I was bewildered that she could be so angry over that.

"Why didn't you lock your car?"

"Well, I trust your neighborhood."

"That's not the point! It's a matter of principle. You must keep your car locked from now on. All this is ignominious."

"What do you mean by that? Are you insulting me?"

"You deserve to be punished; you are evil. Now, come with me and I'll show you what a supposedly educated, refined woman did." She dug her nails in my arms and pushed me outside, then pointed to my car. "You slovenly pig, look how filthy your automobile is. This is my driveway, and if you want to use it, you'd better conform to my rules. Keep your car impeccable, inside and out."

As she approached the car, she continued unloading her blows. "Aren't you ashamed? Look inside. You have newspapers, ugly clothes, and…" she pointed to the back of the car. "Is that chair mine? What are you doing with my chair? Did you steal it from me?"

"That's my chair!"

As she continued to insult me, my indignation mounted and I felt injured by her verbal beating. My resentment was huge. It exasperated me to be offended but unable to say what was on my mind. I wanted to defend myself, but I knew it would do no good. But why did I have to defend myself? There were no rules on how I had to keep my car. I could keep my belongings where I damn well chose without explaining it to anyone. I could keep my car as cluttered as I wanted. Sick or not, she had no right to insult me. And she didn't have the right to go into my car and infringe on my privacy. She brought out the worst in me. I felt blinding rage.

"*Señora,*" I blurted, my lips quivering. "*Lo siento mucho, pero este es mi carro, y solo me concierne a mi como lo mantengo.*"

"I don't understand you," she said. "Speak English or keep your mouth shut."

I was so irritated that I had forgotten to speak English. I took a deep breath and spoke to her in a much calmer tone and enunciated each word. "Come inside. I'll write it down for you."

We went into the living room. I grabbed a piece of paper from the desk and wrote in large print: *I'M SORRY, BUT HOW I KEEP MY BELONGINGS IS MY OWN BUSINESS.*

She read it aloud and shouted, "I should force you to eat your piece of paper! It might be your business how you keep your belongings, but what's done in my house is *my* business. You'd better keep your automobile impeccable or keep it the hell off my property."

I could hardly believe this nightmare was really happening. I struggled to hold back tears. Her words were like a sledgehammer crushing my spirit. Again I resented taking the abuse from her, even if she did have Alzheimer's. Thank God I wasn't in Mexico. If any of my friends were to see me being humiliated this way, they would not believe it. Where was my pride?

I knew I had to leave this madhouse before I ended up like her…bitter and crazy.

I hurried to the bathroom and locked myself in before I did or said anything I would later regret. *To hell with Rafael's and Olivia's advice*, I thought as I splashed water on my face. Finally I pulled myself together, although I was filled with hatred, I prepared her breakfast. I brought the tray to her bedroom and placed it on the night table without saying a word.

"Where is my TV table?" she asked.

"Get it yourself."

I walked out of her room, grabbed my bag, and went to the kitchen for a cup of coffee. As I sipped my coffee I thought on how, as soon as I got home, I would call Mr. Williams to give him back the job of taming his indomitable grandmother. I was done with Mrs. Elizabeth Bromley. This was the last straw, I would definitely quit.

7

Worn-Out

"Good morning, Lolita," Molly said as she entered the kitchen.

I was still fuming but forced myself to smile at her. "Good morning," I said.

"Do you want to talk in the park this morning?" Molly asked kindly.

"No, not today," I said dryly.

"Are you okay? Are you going someplace?"

"I don't feel like talking, Molly. I only want to get out of this miserable place."

"Something's wrong, eh? Maybe I can help—"

The disagreeable voice of Mrs. Bromley interrupted Molly. "Maybe you can help do what?" she asked entering the kitchen.

"Not a big deal, just help with the cooking," Molly said quickly.

"Molly doesn't need any help. And you," she said, pointing to Molly, "take Bowdie out; she's been waiting long enough."

I placed my mug in the sink, picked up my purse, and said, "I'm leaving now."

"Yes, it's time for you to go." Mrs. Bromley paused for a moment and frowned. "Why are you both named Molly?"

Molly shook her head and rolled her eyes. I shrugged and started for the door.

I wanted to shout at her to take a good look at my face—Lolita's face—because she wouldn't see it again.

Since Mr. Williams was unwilling to deal with complaints, I decided I would not give him notice. *Minerva was right; I'm not cut out for this job.*

I rushed to my car. When I got in, staring at me from the passenger seat was "Fighting the Good Fight," a poem from a friend, Ben Tutoli. I picked it up, and although I had read it often, I read it again. This time it had more significance. It was like direction in the midst of uncertainty. I read aloud the lines that touched me the most:

There's the one who fights for prizes

Who gets battered down, but rises.

But the one we eulogize is he or she who
Compromises
And who doesn't come unglued at each rebuff.
And the fact no one denies is
That a corpse, now black with flies, is
The last fool who cries: "I've had enough."
The way survival lies is just to keep on smiling,
Though it is all a bluff.
I reflected on its meaning and felt ashamed of my self-pity. I was reacting childishly, and being self-centered; as if I were the only person in the world going through a rough time. I promised myself that I wouldn't say "I've had enough" again. I would not be battered down; instead, I would rise, and not be a quitter.

When I drove into my driveway, I clicked the remote to open the garage door and prayed for strength, courage and wisdom. I spent the morning doing laundry and straightening up my house. Then I sat down with a cup of coffee and spent some time reading the local newspaper. It all seemed to be bad news and trage-dies, so I set the paper aside and decided to look at my mail, which had been sit-ting on the kitchen counter for a couple of days now due to my unwillingness to deal with it. I opened an official-looking envelope somehow buried under a pile of letters from debt collectors and credit card companies. I felt the blood leaving my head and thought my world would crumble. The notice I dreaded so much was finally here. The bank was going to repossess my property.

That evening, Mrs. Bromley greeted me with a pleasant smile. Then she opened her mouth.

"You look nice," she said, "but your shoes don't match your outfit." She inspected me from head to toe. "Black would be better. Go ahead and change."

"I'm sorry," I said, ignoring her bluntness, "but I don't keep another pair of shoes here."

"Repeat that."

"I said I don't have another pair of shoes here?" I shouted

"*Mon Dieu*! Only peasants and whores wear red shoes."

"But I like them," I said, smiling, when what I wanted was to shut her up. "They're very comfortable."

"I don't care. It's bad taste. Ordinary people wear red, and I don't like ordi-nary people."

"We're not going out, so you're the only one seeing them."

"Well, that's bad enough. It makes me flinch to look at you. And to tell the truth, your skirt is too short. At your age, you should look dignified."

She was at it again. If I ever needed patience, it was now. *Please God, help me ignore her.* "Excuse me, Mrs. Bromley," I said. "I'm going to wash my hands."

"Change your shoes and your skirt too," she yelled as I headed for the bathroom.

I couldn't help but recall the days of my youth with my parents and brothers always criticizing me; and then later my husband always putting me down. I had had enough then, and I didn't intent to go back to the same patron now!

I was determined not to let Mrs. Bromley walk all over me anymore; after all, I had the okay from Mr. Williams to tame her. This was the time to negotiate. She was not going to get any better, and I had made the decision to keep the job. I knew it would take time for me to be able to ignore her insults, but I also knew it was dangerous to build up resentment. If I grew bitter and hateful, it would work against both of us. I just needed deaf ears, and the courage to act on the free license that her grandson granted me to show her who was in charge.

She banged at the door. "What's taking you so long? What're you doing locked in the bathroom?"

"I'm sorry. I have a stomachache."

"It was rude of you to leave while I was still talking."

"I needed to go very badly," I said. What I really wanted was to get away, to calm down and not strangle her where she stood. The bathroom was the perfect place to release the anger building up inside me. I read a couple of magazine articles until I felt relaxed enough to face her again. Surprisingly, she was on her best behavior for the rest of the evening. She looked at my shoes often with a distorted face which seemingly said: *What is this mundane person doing in my prestigious home?*

When bedtime arrived, we said good night and Mrs. Bromley left for her bedroom, Bowdie in toe. I remembered what Olivia had said about the hearing aids squealing, so I followed. As she approached her bedroom I told her I had to fix her hearing aids so they wouldn't speak to her during the night. I didn't know how else to avoid a paranoid rampage. She took the hearing aids out and handed them to me suspiciously. I opened the battery door and placed her aids beside her night table. As I was leaving the room she asked.

"So what did you do to fix them? All I saw you do was open the door."

"Well, yes," I agreed. "But that simple thing will keep them from squealing. Good night, Mrs. Bromley, sleep well." I left the room in a hurry and went to my own room.

A couple of hours later, she showed up at my door, carrying the dog and its bed.

"I want Bowdie to sleep with you tonight."

"What did you say?" I asked incredulously.

"I want Bowdie to sleep with you tonight," she repeated.

"Why on earth do you want her to sleep with me?"

"It's in my will that you'll inherit her." She kissed the dog on its muzzle. "I want my treasure to get used to you; that way, she won't be so devastated when I'm gone. You don't realize the honor I've bestowed upon you."

Obviously she was expecting a round of applause from me.

"What's wrong with you?" she exclaimed. "You're supposed to be thrilled!"

I didn't dare say what I was thinking.

"Come on, don't deny it. You must be beside yourself," she said, followed by a burst of laughter.

I was beside myself but not for the same reason she thought. "I'm really honored by your trust," I lied, "but I'm not used to animals in my room."

"Then it's time you got used to it. Tonight, keep the door closed, so she won't get out. I want her close to you, so she can feel the warmth of your body."

"Not in your life," I mumbled, biting my tongue.

"What did you say?" she asked.

"I said good night, Mrs. Bromley."

"Good night, darling. God bless."

After she left, I wanted to throw the stupid dog against the wall, but the poor thing was not to blame. I would wait until she went to sleep, and take the dog back to her room.

Just when I thought it was safe to leave my room, Mrs. Bromley was back again. "Baby, my baby," she said. "I love you, my angel. You know that, don't you?"

Bowdie jumped out of bed and ran to her. She knelt down and caressed it like a baby. "Believe me, sweetheart," she cooed, "it's a big sacrifice to leave you with Molly, but life is cruel. I might be going to heaven soon to meet with Robert, and you've got to learn how to live without me, like I learned how to live without my dearest Robert."

For a moment, I thought she had come to take the dog back, but my joy was short-lived. She walked over to the bed and placed Bowdie on top of my chest. To my horror, it started licking my face. All I could think about was the cest pool of germs, so I quickly brushed the dog away.

"Why did you do that?" she yelled. "She only wants to kiss you. You are cruel. Aren't you ashamed of yourself?"

"But she's got bad breath."

"That's your fault. You didn't brush her teeth this morning."

I wanted to laugh but kept a straight face. "Yes, Mrs. Bromley, you're right. I'll do it tomorrow."

Bowdie kept licking my face, and I controlled the impulse to hurl the animal across the room. I swallowed my pride and disgust and placed the dog on the bed gently.

"You must take care of her until her time comes, and don't forget to brush her teeth every day. Molly, promise me you will. Go on...promise you will."

I figured it was easier to humor her, so I crossed my fingers and said, "Of course, Mrs. Bromley, I promise."

"*Bon. Bon. Bon nuit,*" she said. She left the room and quietly closed the door behind her. As soon as she had gone, I rushed to the bathroom to wash my face, and then turned on the intercom. When I heard Mrs. Bromley snoring, I took the dog and placed it in its bed next to her.

The next morning, a loud blast from the TV awoke me. Shortly after, Mrs. Bromley pranced into my room, fashionably dressed, with purse in hand. She wore fur-trimmed boots, a beret cocked to one side of her head, and was perfectly done up.

"Well, Bowdie, lazy Molly isn't up yet. Should we wake her? Here we are, ready to leave, and look at her still sleeping."

"No, I'm awake, Mrs. Bromley," I said bolting out of bed. "And where are you going so early and all dressed up?"

"To breakfast," she said, holding the door wide open. "I'm hungry for Virginia ham, bacon, and eggs, because you never cook them."

"You've never asked me to, but I can cook them right now, if you like. We have eggs and—"

"God forbid. I hate the smell of cooking in my house. That's why I eat out every day." She glanced at her watch, and then motioned me to hurry. "I don't like to wait, so hurry up."

"I'll be only a few minutes. Why don't you watch TV in the living room? Meanwhile Molly might get here and she can take you."

"I told you I don't like to wait, so we will leave at this moment. Molly can meet us there. Get moving, I will wait right here."

Afraid she would wander off, I threw on my clothes, not bothering to wash my face, brush my teeth, or even comb my hair.

"Change that dress and those shoes," she said.

"I told you last night that I don't have any extra clothes here."

"There's no point in discussing it any further. You look like a bloody slob."

"For once, I agree with you," I said.

"Aha! You finally know what you are…but there's nothing I can do about it. People are what they are." She shook her finger in my face. "Now, what did you do with my gloves?"

"I haven't seen your gloves."

"Thieves! That's what they are—miserable burglars. They took everything: my money, my jewelry, and all my gloves. I'll put a curse on them." She glared at me and picked up Bowdie.

I was glad she hadn't accused me of the supposed robbery.

As I followed her to the car, I asked, "You do know you can't take her into a restaurant, right?"

"I know that, silly. And don't just stand there—go get a towel for her to sit on my lap."

I rushed into the house, grabbed a towel from the bathroom, and hurried back to the car. I tossed the towel onto her lap and put Bowdie, who growled at me, on her lap. "Where would you like to go?" I asked as I got into the car.

"I don't know. Let's go to any place that serves a decent breakfast."

We drove down Gulf Boulevard, and I stopped at Skidder's, a place known for its delicious breakfast. We left the dog in the car and entered the restaurant.

After the hostess seated us, a waitress came and politely asked, "Ladies, can I get you something to drink?"

"Who's getting in your way? You are mumbling! Speak up." Mrs. Bromley said rudely.

"She's asking if we want something to drink."

I apologized to the waitress and ordered orange juice and coffee for both.

As she left, Mrs. Bromley didn't take her eyes off her.

"Can you guess how old that woman is?" she asked with a little smile.

"No, not really."

"What do you mean, not really?" she snapped. "That woman is too old and too slow to be working in a restaurant." She raised her voice. "Don't you agree?"

I didn't know how to respond to such a comment.

"It's very rude not to answer when I address you, Molly. Do you agree? Yes or no?"

"Maybe that poor woman is like me and has a lot of bills to pay, so she has no other choice," I said, my patience again growing thin.

"Then the both of you should stay at home. It's wrong to work as a waitress at her age."

I took a deep breath and thought of Ben's poem. I prayed I would not come unglued.

"You're very lucky, Molly. You get paid for doing nothing."

Little do you know, I thought. *You are the lucky one. If it weren't for Country-wide Mortgage, I wouldn't have to put up with you.*

The waitress returned and placed the coffees and orange juices on the table. She took out her pad and asked what we wanted.

"Omelet with absolutely no onion. Be very careful because I'm allergic to onion. Do you understand?"

"Yes, I understand."

"Bon. How old are you?" Mrs. Bromley asked.

The woman cleared her throat and said, "Fifty."

Mrs. Bromley looked at her suspiciously. "A very worn-out fifty, I might add."

"Yes, I know," the waitress answered, almost apologetically. "I've had a very hard life. Now, can I get you anything else?"

"No, thank you," I said.

"She is asking me, Molly," Mrs. Bromley said quickly. "I changed my mind, I want ham and eggs, that's why we are here, remember? And don't forget, no onions."

The waitress took my order and left. I looked at Mrs. Bromley straight in the eye. "Do you have fun being cruel?"

"Since when is it cruel to tell the truth?" she sneered.

Embarrassed, I looked at the waitress, who was attending another table. I wished the ground would open up and swallow me. I wanted to apologize on behalf of Mrs. Bromley, but I let it go.

I didn't know what to do to make up for Mrs. Bromley's rude comment. The only thing I could do, given the circumstances, was to leave a twenty-dollar tip. I wished I could have done more.

8

Stark Naked

One Saturday morning, as I was ready to leave, Molly announced, "Lolita, I have an offer that I hope you can't refuse."

"That's my kind of offer. What is it?"

"Would you like to work on Sundays from now on?"

My first reaction was of dismay, promptly followed by excitement at the possibility of earning more money. "Are you asking me in spite of what happened last time?"

"Forget that. I need you on Sundays, starting tomorrow, if it's okay with you."

"So you don't hold against me what I did?" I insisted.

"You didn't do anything. Will you cover Sundays?"

"Yes, Molly, even if it means not going to church anymore," I said, already regretting giving up mass.

"You know, maybe later on you can take her with you to church. She loves to go out and dress up."

"I hope so. I feel guilty about missing mass on Sundays."

I returned that evening with mixed feelings; happy for the extra money but very sad about giving up church.

After supper, I went to the bathroom and took my time scanning a magazine. I was surprised that Mrs. Bromley didn't come to the door to ask what I was doing, as she usually did. Just as I left the bathroom, I was dumbfounded to see her stark naked at my bedroom doorway, holding a handsomely bound book. When she saw me, she went into the room, and I followed her.

Looking defeated, and almost in tears, she said, "Lolita, look at my skin. Once it was as smooth and as white as marble. Why am I like this now? My whole body is a gigantic wrinkle."

I was in shock. Not so much at her nakedness but because she had called me Lolita and not Molly. I felt a stab of pain in my heart for all she had lost, not only

55

her youthful skin, but also her health and her mind. I struggled to find the right words to console her.

"We all go through that," I said finally. "Unfortunately, we can't keep our youthful looks forever."

"Very smart; that's no help at all. Help me get rid of this flabby flesh."

"It's important to keep young at heart and act young. The wrinkles only mean experience and a life well-lived. Each wrinkle represents a memory. Smooth faces have no story behind them. At your age the only thing you can do is to build beauty from the inside out."

She didn't pay any attention to my words but pointed to her legs and her stomach, pinched her arm, and went on, "I'm glad Robert isn't here to see me looking like this."

It was useless to try to comfort her. I tried a different approach. "I admire you," I said. "For your age, you look marvelous—really outstanding," I said, meaning it.

"I hate it when people say 'for your age.' I just want to look good for any age. If you don't have anything clever and believable to say, shut up." She handed me the book she was still holding and smiled kindly, as if trying to make amends for her recent harshness. "Be an angel and tell me when my appointment is."

"Do you have an appointment with your doctor?"

"Yes. Molly made an appointment to have my face done." Then she got closer to me and whispered, "But my family doesn't know, so you'd better don't breathe a word." She kept quiet for a moment, and then added, "My family is mean to me. Nobody cares. You should know by now. They only want my money."

I held the book, wondering if Molly had actually made an appointment with a plastic surgeon. "But that's a big surgery," I said. "Your family should know."

"I'm not asking your opinion," she snarled, baring her teeth. "I'm asking for your help to find the date. Molly wrote it there." She pointed to the book impatiently. "Open the book! Look for it!"

I flipped through December and January and was puzzled to find that Monday, January twenty-six, was circled in red, with the notation: *Dr. Fisherman 9 AM—Face.*

I was dumbfounded. Could she really have an appointment with a plastic surgeon? And if so how did she remember? "Here it is," I said, showing it to her.

"Good," she exclaimed, looking at the date. "But it's a dreadful wait." She patted her cheeks, and then grabbed her breasts. "I'll ask Molly to take me to the doctor right away. First, my face—later, my body."

"I'm happy for you," I said.

In reality, I was concerned. I definitely planned to discuss this with Molly on Monday.

"Mrs. Bromley," I said, "don't you think you should cover yourself up? You don't want to catch a cold."

"*Mon Dieu*, you are right. I could die of pneumonia. I need to be healthy to have my face done. I really don't mind if I die, you know, but I want to die looking the way I used to look." She looked at herself in the mirror and moved her head from side to side. "How terrible; I look awful." She tapped her image in the mirror and said, "Elizabeth, you must look glamorous when you meet with Robert; he admired your beauty so much." She closed her eyes. With a self-satisfied grin, she continued, "Oh, Lolita, he showed me off all over the world and showered me luxuriously with everything money could buy." She leaned toward me, lowering her voice. "But he never, ever touched me. Can you believe that?"

"What do you mean, he never touched you?"

"Exactly that! He never made love to me." She looked up and placed her hands together, as if in prayer. "Oh, Robert, my love, why couldn't you?"

"Will you please get dressed?" I asked impatiently.

"Don't you find it strange? He adored my looks."

"Get dressed, please," I insisted.

"He did love me. Why, then, couldn't he get it up? God knows I tried!"

"Please, Mrs. Bromley, it's cold. Put your nightgown on. Go to your room."

She left, and my heart went out to her. She sounded defeated; there was not a trace of her usual arrogance. Seeing her like that diminished the grudge I held against her. I knew that Mrs. Bromley's wrinkles were the least of her problems.

It saddened me to think of the future awaiting her.

I hopped into bed and thought about former president, Ronald Reagan, when he was stricken by this treacherous illness. I now understood better how sad he must have felt when, knowing of his disease, he had addressed the nation in his farewell speech. I admired Nancy Reagan, who had promised to stay at his side to see him through the long and lonely journey.

The image of beautiful Rita Hayworth also came to mind. When I had first heard the news that she suffered from Alzheimer's, I hadn't known anything about the disease. Knowing now how devastating the illness is, I thought how lucky Rita was to have her daughter Jasmine caring for her while drifting away into the lonely journey to nowhere.

It took me a long time to fall asleep, and when I finally did, Mrs. Bromley's high-pitched voice woke me up.

"Molly," she said, "be an angel and help me find my baby girl."

"I'm sure she is somewhere in the house. Don't worry."

"Somewhere? Yes, that much I know. But where, damn it? Is looking for her too much to ask?"

"Of course not." I answered, trying to be agreeable.

We searched every room and every corner of the house until finally I gave up.

"We'll look for Bowdie tomorrow."

"Tomorrow? Are you out of your mind? I'll die if we don't find my baby tonight."

I had no other choice but to continue the search. I went over the same places we had already been. Finally, I entered her bedroom again and heard scratching inside the bathroom. When I opened the door, Bowdie came running out.

"You are smarter than you look. You found my jewel. I owe you one. Some mean person must have locked her in there. I insist that you find out who did such an atrocious thing. You must investigate!"

"Tomorrow I'll investigate," I said.

I chuckled all the way to my bedroom.

Early Sunday morning, I awoke to a loud moaning. I found Mrs. Bromley hunched over, sitting in the living room.

"What's wrong?"

"This pain is killing me!" she cried, holding her right arm.

"Let me get you a painkiller," I said, stroking her shoulder lightly. I rushed to the kitchen.

"Please, hurry! I can't take this anymore! I'm a good person. Why does God punish me this way? Robert, take me, I'm ready…I don't want to suffer anymore. It's more than I can endure. Robert, don't waste time. Hurry up. Take me right now."

I grabbed the ibuprofen and Stopain spray. When I came closer, her lament became louder. "God, Oh God, are you punishing me for my sins? I swear I have never hurt anyone intentionally."

"Please, take these pills." I handed her a glass of water. After she had swallowed them, I explained, "The pills will take time to work, but now I'm going to spray your arm with this. It works right away. It'll feel very cold, but the pain will go away at once." I repeated it so she would be prepared, but as I started to spray the Stopain, she slapped the can away, sending it flying across the room.

"Bloody stupid woman! That's ice-cold!" she screamed at the top of her lungs.

Although I wanted to throw the can back at her, I counted to ten to give myself time to calm down, and picked it up. "Your pain will go away sooner with this," I said in a soothing tone.

"That's what you think, stupid!"

"Please, watch your tongue. I'll be in my room, in case you need me." I said, leaving her alone to deal with her arthritis pain.

And that was the way I began Sunday.

Once in my room, I watched mass on TV and hoped for a peaceful day.

Later, I prepared breakfast and took the tray to her bed. She smiled charmingly and said, "Thank you, darling Molly."

I left her bedroom annoyed because she insisted on calling me Molly; I felt like I was being robbed of my identity, once more.

By noon, she was still in bed. I took advantage of my solitude and meditated contemplating nature's beauty. I stood by the dining room's sliding glass door, gazing out at the fish jumping in the quiet water, boats gliding across the bay, and blue herons still as statues standing on several tree's trunks. I was sad and felt cut off from the world. Once more, I felt trapped. I recalled the many times I'd had the same feeling. I wondered why, when I was surrounded by beautiful, peaceful surroundings, I had this frustrating turmoil inside. I remembered the time my husband and I went for a long trip to Spain on our honeymoon. I was thrilled to cross the ocean with a man who had swept me off my feet and who promised to show me the world. But soon my dream became a nightmare when I discovered the dark side of my brand-new husband.

The journey on the Italian cruise ship Michelangelo lasted ten days of constant arguments. We were most of the time inside the cabin, arguing. I spent the early mornings reading the ship's program, which intensified my frustration, for it made me aware of what I was missing while being a prisoner in a jail without bars.

We disembarked in Barcelona on a cold January afternoon. Upon arriving at the luxurious Grand Hotel, its charm made me gasp with admiration. I set out to forget the bad moments lived during the sailing and prepared for a real honeymoon—I felt like Cinderella. It was a short-lived dream because as soon as we entered the suite, Mauricio made plans to have all meals delivered to the suite. I felt his prisoner once again.

He hated stores and crowds, so any shopping was done from the room. I would gladly have traded the time I spent in that magnificent hotel suite for just one day in an ordinary department store. I longed to walk along the streets lined with thick beautiful trees and colorful boutiques. When traveling abroad I expected to mingle with the townspeople, compare accents, and learn about the folklore of the country. I found it unbearable to be locked up inside a hotel—no matter how luxurious—while outside on the open all sorts of people were doing their will. The uncertainty of ever going back to Spain burned inside me.

Mauricio occasionally went out for business meetings but demanded that I wait for him in the room. Sometimes I did, but sometimes I sneaked out, making sure to be back before him. I used to walk along *La Rambla de las Flores* until I knew it by heart. But because of my escapades, I was less frustrated when I welcomed him in the evening.

He didn't allow me to go to mass. Instead, we spent all day in bed making love until I ended up hating it.

One Sunday, I was fed up with sex and with him, so I pulled away, shouting, "Leave me alone!"

"What's wrong with you? Any woman would die to be in your place."

"I'm fed up with sex. I want a break."

"Are you frigid? Is that it?"

"Think what you want, but leave me alone. You're obsessed with sex."

"You lied to me; you made me believe you were a passionate woman. You'll cry blood when you lose me. What the hell else do you want, when you have everything?"

"Freedom! Companionship! I'm sick and tired of being locked up and waiting for you to come back and satiate your animal needs!" I shouted, running away from the room, thinking how different everything would have been if my brilliant, wealthy husband were human.

"Lolitaaa! Where are you?" Mrs. Bromley shouted, bringing me back from my memories.

"I'm here, Mrs. Bromley," I answered, stepping into her bedroom.

"What time is it?" she asked.

"One-thirty."

"Is it day or night?"

"It's afternoon, Mrs. Bromley."

"Did I eat lunch?"

"Not yet."

"In that case, I'll be ready in half an hour," she said, getting out of bed.

"Do you feel okay now? No more pain?"

"Pain? Why? Should I have any pain?"

"Well, you were in pain this morning."

She looked at me with a puzzled expression. "Pain? You must be taking me for someone else."

Sometime later, during lunch at Red Lobster, she ordered a double scotch on the rocks.

"Mrs. Bromley, that's too strong. Don't you want to mix it with soda? You shouldn't drink on an empty stomach."

"I know what I want, and how I like it. You ask for whatever you want and leave me alone."

I quickly asked the waitress to bring something to munch on. Mrs. Bromley didn't touch the peanuts and cheese but finished her scotch and asked for a second one.

She kept staring at some children sitting across from us; I hoped she wouldn't bother them.

"I don't know why people bring children to restaurants," she said loudly.

Heads turned in our direction, and I wished I had wings to fly away.

"She went on. "They should eat at home and let the grown-ups eat in peace."

"Please, don't talk so loudly. Everybody is looking at you," I whispered.

"What did you say?" she shouted.

I grabbed a piece of paper from my purse and printed: *YOU ARE SPEAKING TOO LOUD.*

"Am I? I'm so sorry. You should have told me."

She was quiet for a while, and then one of the children across from us knocked over a glass of milk. The boy began to cry.

Mrs. Bromley deliberately addressed the mother. "Do you see what you get for bringing children to public places? They should stay at home and not bother others."

I went over to the child and said, "Don't cry, honey. Accidents can happen to anyone. That lady is a sick person. She really doesn't mean what she says."

I turned to the mother and apologized for Mrs. Bromley.

This, and the last incident, when she was so mean to the waitress, made me think about the saying: "Be careful what you wish for; you might get it." One of the reasons why I had wanted the day shift was because of the opportunity to eat out. Now I wondered if I still wanted to work in the daytime and eat out every day.

9

Clinton-Monica

It amazed me how trivial incidents would send Mrs. Bromley into a combat mode.

One Saturday evening, I arrived a few minutes late, to find her waiting by the gate. Molly was in her car, and when she saw me, she waved good-bye and drove away.

"How dare you keep me waiting, Molly? You're very late."

"I'm sorry," I said. "There was a problem on the bridge."

"I've had it!" she shouted, with a look on her face that frightened me. "I pay people to do things right, but instead, everything is done wrong! Molly, you neglected me! My grandson will hear about this, oh yes, he will!"

She walked into the kitchen and thrusted the phone into my hand. "Here, dial. I want to talk to Gary immediately. Things have to change around here, or I'll disinherit him."

I placed my purse on the counter then called my home, and left a message in my answering machine. I told her, "He's not there, but I left a message on his machine. I'm sure he'll call you as soon as he gets back."

"I'll hold you responsible, so you'd better call again and again until you find him; otherwise, I'll put the evil eye on you. Do you hear?"

"Yes, Mrs. Bromley."

"I'm not happy here. I hate this house."

"I thought you loved your home. It's a nice house." I said.

"I don't like anything around here, and I especially don't like you, or the way you do things." She opened a drawer. "Look at the silverware. It's not in order. And my Wedgwood doesn't look good over there, and the lighting of the paintings is wrong. Nothing works since you came here."

"Mrs. Bromley, I'm only your night companion, not your maid," I dared say. "I'm here only to look after you."

"That's no way to talk to me." She pushed my shoulder. "You're bloody disrespectful. Besides being a thief, you are lazy."

I turned a deaf ear. Finally, I was learning not to listen.

One afternoon, while we were having a pleasant time, we heard a noise from outside my bedroom window.

"What's going on out there?" she asked, going into my bedroom.

"I don't know," I said, following her.

As she stepped inside, she grabbed her head. "What the bloody hell is this?" she shouted, pointing to a pile of magazines and books on my bed. "What a disgusting pigsty! I will not tolerate this disorder in my home. I don't know how I'm able to put up with your filthy habits. When will you learn to be neat like me?"

I marveled at the speed with which she could change from likeable to hateful in a second. I felt so confused looking into her eyes. Why couldn't I understand what was deep down behind those eyes? It was difficult for me at these times to remember Rafael's advice and Ben's poem. I had to try harder to ignore her. I removed everything from my bed, and she calmed down.

"Lolitaaaa! Come quickly, immediately," Mrs. Bromley called from the living room.

"Yes?" I asked, rushing to her side, my heart pounding.

"Can you explain why there is so much ado about a cigar?"

"What do you mean?"

"Clinton and Monica. Is Clinton our president?"

"Yes."

"Is Monica the first lady? Were they caught smoking in the oval office?"

"Not exactly."

"Not exactly? What kind of a bloody answer is that? Not exactly she is not the first lady, or not exactly they weren't smoking?"

"Well…neither." She gave me an exasperated look.

Mrs. Bromley wanted to be up to date regarding the Bill Clinton and Monica Lewinsky scandal, and she followed the news closely on television. I explained—and she forgot. She always began with simple questions and we ended up in heated argument.

I dreaded watching the news with her, because she asked the same questions over and over again. I wished the scandal were over. When I changed the channel to watch *Family Feud*, she insisted on watching the news about Clinton's scandal.

"I don't understand why the media is crucifying the poor man just because Monica smoked a cigar in the oval office. Who cares about a cigar? Maybe they meant something else. What do you think?"

"I don't know anything about it."

"So what's new, my dear? You never know anything about anything. I don't know how you survive in life."

"It's teatime," I said, jumping to my feet. "I'll be back soon."

"At least that's something you know how to make."

I was back in a few minutes with a pot of tea and two mugs.

"Change my mug," she said. "I hate thick rims. Use good china. And I told you to cover your head when working in the kitchen. I don't like hair in my food."

I took a deep breath and showed my sweetest smile while answering, "Dear Mrs. Bromley, I'm not your maid. Do you agree?"

I expected a blow; instead she replied with a sweet smile, "Sometimes I like you. Your expression does not match your disrespectful words. You must not be that dumb."

I burst into laughter and went to the dining room for a china cup. When I returned, she said, "Tell me about Clinton."

I didn't answer.

"Did you hear me?"

"He had an affair," I managed to say.

"An affair? So what? Affairs are as old as passion and lust," she said, with a mischievous smile.

"So what?" I repeated. "He's a married man."

"Big deal! All married men cheat."

"For heaven's sake, Mrs. Bromley, he needs to set an example. Not only is he a married man, but he's the president of the United States."

"But he's still a man with temptations. Blood runs through his veins." She grinned. "And hot blood, if you ask me."

"He could have waited to finish his term," I added.

"Oh, you naïve woman. Let the man have his thrills when he feels the urge, and not a century later." She laughed, as if amused by her own words.

"Mrs. Bromley, you seem to know a lot about life, so why do you need to ask me?"

"I want to know who smoked that bloody cigar and why the media does not let up on it." She shook a finger at me. "You ought to know who smoked that cigar. Say something! Speak your mind! I want to have an intelligent conversation with you."

She made so much sense that it confused me. I wished I were able to figure out how her mind worked. She could be so lucid at times and so deranged at others.

"Lolita, will you please come back from limbo? Can we have a decent conversation? I want to know everything about those two."

It pleased me that she used my own name.

"Of course we can, Mrs. Bromley. Since I'm entitled to my own opinion, I say Clinton shouldn't have used the Oval Office for his shady business."

"And my opinion," she said, with a frown, "is that he was smart using his own territory." She took a sip of tea. "This is cold. And why? Because you didn't put the cozy on the teapot, and now it's bloody cold. But never mind—I can't expect good service from you. Monica...is that her name? Maybe she didn't even smoke the cigar. Giving it another thought, maybe she smoked his private part instead. I'm pretty sure he said that they didn't have intercourse, so I'll bet she gave him a mighty good—how do Americans say—blow job. Don't you think?"

I was shocked. To my chagrin, I felt like I had to laugh.

"What is your opinion on the blow job?"

Before I would burst out laughing, I picked up the tray and said, "I'll make you some hot tea."

"You didn't answer me. Are you for the blow job or not!"

"I'll be back," I said, and rushed to the kitchen.

As I reheated the tea, I could hear her yelling, "Answer me!"

"I can't hear you!" I yelled back.

She appeared in the kitchen. "Well, Miss Lolita, have you ever given a blow job? Did you like it? Were you good at it?"

"Blow jobs were not my forte, so I couldn't say." Then, in an attempt to change the subject, I asked, "Do you know if your grandson is coming over to see you tonight?" I marched back to the living room, carrying the tray.

She followed me. "If you don't answer, I'll ask Gary," she said.

"Change the subject, will you? I'm sick of the whole Clinton event." I said.

"Who do you think you are? I'm the one choosing topics. If you have a problem talking about sex, you must be frigid, but that's your business. I'll ask Gary what I want to know, and I'll also accuse you of lack of knowledge, plus being a boring companion."

"I'm really sorry if I fail to amuse you," I said, trying to appease her.

"You can't help being who you are. Now, it's time to draw the drapes."

"Mrs. Bromley," I said, "can we keep them open a little longer?" I always thought it was a pity to shut out such a magnificent view.

"Why?"

"To watch the sunset," I said, smiling.

"I don't care about sunsets," she sneered.

"But I do. I always watch them from my house. It never ceases to amaze me when the sky lights up with such spectacular afterglow of colors."

Mon Dieu! How trite! Go on, then, and watch whatever you want from your own house. I don't give a damn about bloody trivialities."

I mentally sent her to hell, but I was quickly sorry and prayed for a miraculous change in her attitude, not only for my sake, but for hers and that of others who would cross her path. Was this Alzheimer's talking or was she just a mean-spirited. Does Alzheimer's impair kindness? I took a deep breath and thought that life is unfair, and some illnesses just don't believe in miracles.

That night, in bed, I reflected on my life. I understood that Mrs. Bromley's nastiness was because of her sickness; but had my husband been sick when he put me through hell? His constant criticism had crushed my spirit. I wondered why I attracted the same kind of personality. My father had been a tyrant and had marked my youth; my husband had ruined my adult life, and now Mrs. Bromley was spoiling my golden years. Did I unconsciously allow them to do that to me?

I had always hated Sundays because it was the saddest day of the week when I was married. This Sunday, around noon, I was waiting for Mrs. Bromley to finish dressing to go to lunch.

We met in the vestibule. "I can't find my gloves," she said good-naturedly. "Be an angel and find them for me."

I reassured her once more. "You don't need gloves in Florida. Mrs. Bromley, you don't have any."

"What? I have dozens of leather gloves. Somebody must have stolen them. I'll place a curse on all of them. They'll perish." She paused and stared at my dress.

"Why are you wearing that bloody thing?"

Oh lord, not again, I thought. *Why doesn't she leave me alone?* "What's wrong with it? I think it's pretty. In fact, it's one of my favorites."

"You have too many bright colors; too young-looking. Tell me, do you enjoy calling attention to yourself?"

In the name of God, how can this old hag keep at it in such a manner? I thought how wonderful it would be if I were walking on the beach, far away from her and her awful criticism.

"Well? Did you hear me?"

I sighed. "Yes, I heard you."

"Do you like men looking at you as if you were offering your flesh in a meat market? Yes? No?"

"What kind of a question is that? Of course not."

"Then use conservative solid colors. Go ahead and change into black, or navy, even gray. And cover up that cleavage."

"I'm sorry, but I don't keep other clothes here."

"I hate people wearing mine, but I'll make an exception." She walked toward her bedroom. "Come on, look in my wardrobe and try on whatever suits you."

I didn't follow her. "Very kind of you, Mrs. Bromley, but I hate to wear other people's clothes."

"You should feel flattered by my offer."

"Oh, I do. I really appreciate your generosity."

"I don't think you do. *C'est la vie.* Let's go." With her nose up in the air, she headed out the front door.

We went to Red Lobster, and since it was crowded, I got her some wine while we waited for a table in the bar. A hostess gave us a vibrating pager.

"What is this thing?" Mrs. Bromley asked.

"It tells you when your table is ready."

"I want to hold it."

I gave her the pager.

"Something's wrong with this," she said a few seconds later. "I can't feel anything."

"Be patient. It'll happen soon."

"We are going to miss the call. This is taking too long. Somebody will take our table."

"Be patient. Enjoy your drink and forget about it."

Without warning, Mrs. Bromley flung the pager and her drink across the room, nearly hitting an elderly couple.

"What the bloody hell is this?" she shouted.

Her reaction stunned and embarrassed me. Why did she have to behave like this? Nevertheless, I tried to calm her down. "Don't worry, dear. It's only an accident."

The hostess rushed over and picked up the pager from the floor, then escorted us to a booth while a busboy swept up the broken glass.

Soon after, a young waitress came over to our table.

"Have you decided what you want?"

While the waitress wrote our order for lunch, Mrs. Bromley stared at the girl's hands, "Do you really like those nails?"

"They're cool," the girl answered with pride. "Do you like them?"

"Goodness gracious, no. I hate them. They're for streetwalkers, not for a pretty young girl like you." She reached for the girl's hand. "*Mon Dieu*, look at those long, square, green, disgusting nails."

The girl smiled sweetly, "That's exactly what my grandmother said, but all my friends love them."

"Ignorant generation! Mature people know better. We have good taste."

"I'll tell my grandmother what you said," the waitress said, still smiling. "I'll be back in a sec with your drinks."

We had our wine. We were toasting each other when three men, following the hostess, passed by and sat a few tables away from us. Mrs. Bromley stared at them. "Look at him," she said, pointing a finger at their table. "How rude. He did not remove his hat. That's unacceptable."

"You're being rude yourself by pointing. Please don't stare at them," I said emphatically, dreading what she might do next.

"What?" she shouted. I quickly produced a piece of paper from my purse and wrote: DO NOT STARE AT THOSE MEN.

"I'm entitled to look wherever I wish," she replied in a shrill voice as she drummed her fingers on the table.

"It's the same thing with that man," I said. "He's entitled to wear his hat."

"Pardon?" she asked, moving closer to me. "What did you say?"

"Nothing important," I replied, not wanting to raise my voice.

"If it's not important, why did you say it?"

I cleared my throat and took a sip from my drink.

The waitress came back with our lunch, but I had lost my appetite and forced myself to eat a little. Later, she came back and read the dessert choices.

"I'd like chocolate cheesecake, please," Mrs. Bromley said, "but first I want you to be kind and tell that man over there to be a gentleman and take off his hat."

The waitress looked surprised. "Excuse me, ma'am?"

Mrs. Bromley stared at her. "It's poor manners to wear a hat indoors. Well, don't just stand there, young lady. Go over there!"

"I'm very sorry," the waitress said, her smile frozen. "I can't do that. He's a customer, just like you."

"Well if you can't, I'll tell him myself."

I jumped to my feet. "Mrs. Bromley, if you do that, I will leave at once and leave you alone here." Her eyes narrowed, pushed me aside and walked toward the men's table.

Since I couldn't leave the restaurant without her, I stood up gingerly and took refuge in the ladies' room. I splashed water on my face and waited a few minutes dreading what awaited me. I braced myself for the worst and walked out of the bathroom.

I glanced at their table. The men were grinning, standing in front of a radiant Mrs. Bromley, engrossed in a conversation. I sighed with relief and returned to my table.

The man, with the hat still on, escorted her back. He bowed and said something in French to me, then with a polite bow, kissed Mrs. Bromley's hand. "*Merci beaucoup, madame*," he said.

"*Au revoir, monsieur*," she replied with an engaging smile. Her eyes followed him as he returned to his table.

"What happened, Mrs. Bromley?" I asked, full of curiosity.

"Oh, what charming men! They don't speak English, so I translated the menu for them," she said proudly.

"How nice of you," I said, relieved. "What happened? The man is still wearing his hat."

"Sad, very sad. The poor gentleman had brain surgery and his head is covered with scars. He's in the process of healing."

As we drove home Mrs. Bromley was enveloped in her thoughts and I in mine. I recalled a similar occurrence while living in Spain. We had rented an apartment in Barcelona with a spectacular view of Montserrat. Mauricio used one of the rooms as his office. One day, a businessman came to visit.

"*Señor* Melero, this is Lolita, my wife," Mauricio said, as he introduced me.

The man turned to me, bowed politely, and took my hand to his lips. "It is a pleasure to meet such a beautiful young *señora*."

"What do you think you are doing kissing my wife's hand?" Mauricio shouted.

"It's the gesture of a *caballero* to kiss a lady's hand," he answered calmly.

"Where's the gentleman? I don't see one."

"I am a *caballero*. You are insulting me."

"A *caballero*? You are in my home, in front of my wife, and you have not removed your hat. Do you call that being a gentleman?"

"Lolita," Mrs. Bromley said, bringing me back from my short trip to the past. "Before we get home, do you think we need to stop for groceries?"

"I don't think so."

"Good. We'll go straight home to my adorable baby."

"Bowdie's fine, don't worry. Now, Mrs. Bromley, what else did you find out about the man with the hat?"

"What man? What hat? What are you talking about?"

The fleeting moments of lucidity were gone. I hadn't asked right away, so I had missed the opportunity to learn more about the French men. I thought that it would be a blessing to erase from your memory the things that brought grief—but how terrible it would be not to be able to recall those that brought happiness.

I recalled an article I had read recently about the mentally ill, senile, alcoholics, and children; nothing restrains them from saying what comes to mind. Society forbids us from saying to others what we really think. Mrs. Bromley no longer had the mind to know what to keep to herself. I pondered this, wrapped in a sea of sadness, brought on by the realization of Mrs. Bromley's incapacity to discern.

10

Eye Surgery

Molly was waiting for me as I arrived one Friday evening.

"I need to talk to you right now," she said. "I forgot to tell you that Mrs. Bromley's having eye surgery early Monday morning." She handed me a small bottle. "Be sure to put a drop in the left eye every hour, starting Sunday night at six, until she goes to bed, and then again when she wakes up in the morning. Please have her ready to go at seven, and don't let her eat or drink anything."

"Okay, but what about the face-lift?" I asked.

"It will be done on the twenty-sixth."

"Two surgeries in one month? Won't that be too much at her age?"

"Apparently not. She's in perfect health," Molly answered.

"I know, she's as strong as a mule and twice as ornery," I said. We both laughed. Then I asked, "What about her medicine for nerves?"

Molly paused for a moment. "Give her double Kava 55. No, you better make it six pills Sunday night."

"I think that's too much?"

"Kava's natural. It won't hurt her."

"What are you two talking about out there?" Mrs. Bromley shouted from the front door.

Molly jumped in her car. "Good luck, Lolita!" she yelled, pulling out. "You'll need it."

Monday morning Mrs. Bromley was ready when Molly arrived at seven, and they left for the hospital without incident. Shortly after, I left for my home and took Bowdie with me.

When I returned that evening, Molly was in the kitchen. "How was the surgery?" I asked. "How's Mrs. Bromley?"

"It didn't happen," Molly replied. "The old gal is fine."

"What do you mean?"

"Well, when she didn't recognize her own doctor, he wanted me to obtain authorization from her family in order to perform the surgery."

"So did you ask them?"

"No, but I took her to see her lawyer. He drew me a power of attorney."

"So what's next?" I asked.

"Since I have the power of attorney, the doctor will take her tomorrow."

"Should I do the eye drop every hour tonight?"

"Yeah. Same. And have her ready at seven."

"What am I going to do at seven?" Mrs. Bromley said from the kitchen doorway.

"We're debating about your medicine," Molly said.

"I don't know what you are saying."

Molly escorted her to the bedroom. When Molly came back a short time later, she whispered, "What I'd really like to give her is arsenic."

"Just tell me when and I'll help you get it," we laughed.

That evening, after Mrs. Bromley was in bed, her grandson called.

"Hi, Lolita. How are you doing?"

"I'm fine, thanks."

"How's my grandmother?"

"She's doing fine."

"Her eye is not hurting her?"

"Then you don't know?"

"Know what?" he asked.

"She didn't have the surgery."

"What? Why?"

"I'm not sure, but it seems that she was confused, and the doctor asked Molly for written authorization. Molly went to the lawyer and got a power of attorney, and they—"

"What?" he yelled. "Molly can't have power of attorney." He paused for a moment. "Listen, Lolita, I'll be there in the morning to pick up my grandmother. I'll call Molly now and tell her to meet me at the hospital."

Something was very wrong; I could tell by the tone of his voice. I didn't understand why Molly hadn't called Mr. Williams or Jane. And I wondered why she had taken it upon herself to see the attorney, when calling Mr. Williams or Jane would have sufficed. This situation had me tossing and turning all night because I trusted Molly. In the morning, Mr. Williams picked up his grandmother, and I left with Bowdie.

Upon my return in the afternoon, I found Molly vacuuming the carpet in the dining room.

"How come you aren't ready to leave?"

She turned the machine off. "Mrs. Bromley knocked over a vase of flowers, so I wanted to clean up before I left."

"Did Mr. Williams call you last night?"

"Yeah, and he was pretty upset with me. What I'd like to know is how he found out I got the power of attorney. Do you know anything about it?"

I felt guilty and wished I hadn't opened my big mouth, but my obligation was to Mr. Williams—and he had asked me what happened. But I didn't want to get her in trouble. "I thought he knew."

"No, he didn't." She picked up a few flowers from the floor and turned to me. "I didn't think it was that important, and now he's treating me like dirt."

"I hope you're not upset with me. I wouldn't want to mess things up for you."

"I'm not mad at you, Lolita. I'm mad at the whole world. I'm fed up with Mr. Williams, Jane, and the whole damn job."

"Molly!" Mrs. Bromley shouted as she came into the room. "Are you talking about my grandson?" She sat down and adjusted the patch over her eye.

"Yes," Molly answered. "Don't you remember how angry he was with me this morning? He thinks I'm plotting to get your money, but I only tried to help by showing him how efficient I was, and—"

Mrs. Bromley cut in, "But we know *he is* the one after my money. He sold my land in Canada, my properties, my jewelry…he dispersed my fortune. Now put that bloody sweeper away and take care of my tea."

Molly smiled, looped the cord around the vacuum cleaner, and stood it in a corner. "Lolita will get your tea. I have to leave now. Ask her for anything you want." Molly turned to me and whispered, "Don't give her scotch tonight. Make it a Virgin Mary instead."

"Molly, how dare you whisper about me with a stranger?"

"Lolita's not a stranger. She takes care of you when I'm not here."

"Who is Lolita?"

Molly grinned. "I mean the other Molly, and remember how nicely she prepares your tray. Just the way you like it."

"I do not care. I pay you to be here. I want you, not Molly. Don't leave me alone with that person. I think she is the one my grandson hired to spy on me. I do not want anybody in my house but you."

I tried to relieve her worries. "Oh, no, Mrs. Bromley," I said. "I would never spy on you. I'm here to help Molly take care of you. We don't want you alone, ever."

"Come on, now." Molly said, helping Mrs. Bromley back to the sofa. "Lolita—I mean, Molly—takes good care of you." She turned to me. "Don't pay attention to what she says. She's confused because of the sedative."

Mrs. Bromley picked up a photograph of her dead husband from the end table. "Uh, um…Robert, *mon amour*," she said, her eyes riveted on the image. "I do not want to stay alone with that woman." She turned to Molly and pointed at me. "Do not leave me with that stranger. I will give you all the money you want, but stay with me."

"You'll be safe with Lolita."

Mrs. Bromley looked at Molly with a straight face, "Do you think I can trust her? Is she smart, witty, clever?" She placed the picture back on the table and stared at me.

Molly winked at me and said, "Of course she's all of that, and more. Besides, she likes you."

Mrs. Bromley reached for Molly's arm and whispered loud enough for me to hear, "*Entre nous*, does she have black blood in her?"

I laughed out loud.

Molly was quick to answer, "No, but she does have a beautiful tan."

Mrs. Bromley eyed me carefully. "Molly, I don't want a stupid, boring person keeping me company. Do you hear?"

I walked over and sat next to her; I placed my hand on her arm, but she brushed it away. I smiled as I gazed into her eyes, wishing to reassure her. "Mrs. Bromley, I really do care about you."

"Really? Do you?"

"Really. I do."

"Was Robert with me while I had surgery?" she asked, with a deep sigh and downcast look. I tried to sound convincing when I ventured to say, "I'll bet he's hovering over you right now—and always, whenever you need him. You must have faith." It saddened me to see the fear, confusion and deep sadness in her face. "I have an idea Mrs. Bromley. Would you like to play a game?" I asked.

"Play a game?" She repeated. "Are you not too old for games?"

"We are never too old for games. Listen, I have heard all these stories about you being such a talented dancer when you lived in Paris. Let's pretend I am a reporter from the *Paris Match* and you granted me a one time interview. Will you do it?"

"Oh my, how intriguing," she said with a new spark in her eye.

"OK. So you granted me an interview. While I prepare your tea you think about the interview and what you are going to say."

I went to the kitchen to prepare her tea and when I came back, tray in hand, I found her entering the living room clad in a wide-brimmed hat, green gardening gloves and wearing bright, red lipstick.

I almost dropped the tray.

"Who are you?" she asked bewildered

"My name is Ginger. I am with the *Paris Match*, I was sent to interview you."

"*Bon, entrez s'il vous plait, asseyez vous.*"

"Mrs. Bromley, excuse me, I am from the English branch of the *Paris Match*, I don't speak French."

"I am so sorry dear. Not to worry, I am British myself, so I speak English. Go on, have a seat," she said, as she sat on the antique chair.

I placed the tea tray by her side.

"How delightful!" she declared.

I grabbed a notepad and pen from the kitchen and sat ready to take notes.

I began with, "Madam Bromley, do you remember the name of the places you danced in Paris?"

"How could I forget?" Her expression became free from tension, a little smile bloomed on her lips conveying a sweetness I hadn't seen before. "The stage was my life…The Lido, Maxim, Follies Bergerec…I can still hear the applause and see me bowing graciously for the audience. The "interview" went on for almost one hour and I was amazed to hear her talk about events and dates as if they had happened yesterday. A happy grin never left her face and I felt great satisfaction. We sat in silence next to each other for a short while when she leaned toward me and said. "You know, you are smart after all…I think I might grow to like you."

Molly appeared distressed when she arrived the next morning. She took Bowdie to the park without her usual smile.

On my way home, after I had driven several blocks, Molly's sad face haunted me. I thought that if I talked to her it would help, so I decided to go back to the park. She was standing near the water when I approached her.

Her face brightened. "I thought you had gone."

"You looked worried this morning so I turned back. Is there anything I can do?"

"Thanks, but there's nothing anyone can do," she sighed. "Let me get Bowdie so we can chat. Let's sit over there on that bench." She tied the dog close to her.

"I couldn't sleep last night," she said. "I thought about what Mr. Williams said to me." She caught a tear. "Lolita, he's wrong. He said I had ulterior motives, but I swear I didn't."

"But Molly, maybe you should have called him before doing anything."

"You know, when the doctor told me that we needed that paper, I thought of Mrs. Bromley's lawyer. I met him several times when I took her to see him. That's why we went to his office for advice. Mrs. Bromley acted very sound when she asked him for the power of attorney. Of course, it was restricted to only that one time. I only wanted to prove to Mr. Williams that I could solve a problem without bothering him."

"But you should have had a member of the family there, and then you wouldn't have needed that paper."

"I was in charge of her," Molly said. "She was my responsibility."

"But Mr. Williams is her closest family, and he is our boss."

"Mrs. Bromley is my boss," she said.

"Nevertheless, Molly, we are supposed to report anything important to him, or to Jane."

I didn't agree with Molly. I knew Mrs. Bromley was not capable of making any important decisions on her own.

Molly was adamant. "Mrs. Bromley pays me with her own money. I only answer to her."

"Listen, Molly, I know it's not my business, but since she suffers from dementia, we owe Mr. Williams a detailed report of everything that's out of routine. Why don't you talk with him again, and maybe even with Jane? Clear the air."

"I don't like her. I know I didn't do anything wrong, and they're free to think whatever they want." She smiled, "And I don't think Mrs. Bromley's that sick." She placed her hand on my arm. "Disoriented, yes; senile?—not yet. I know she's still able to manage her money, but they took that pleasure away from her. The poor woman's right: they don't care about her."

"Molly, you could be wrong. Mr. Williams spends a small fortune on his grandmother. He could hire cheaper help; instead, he wants the best."

"Lolita, don't you forget that it's her money he is spending, not his."

"Still, he could spend less on her and have more money for himself."

"You don't know what I know. I don't agree with what they're doing to her, that's all."

"Look at you! You're so upset. For your own sake, talk to them and get it off your chest."

"I'll think about it. Anyhow, I'm fed up with this job and I do worry when I see how little they care about Mrs. Bromley. She unburdens herself with me, and I get depressed because I care for her. I don't need that."

I knew I wasn't making any progress. I said, "I don't know what to tell you. I haven't been here long enough to judge anything or anyone."

"I'm here all day and I've been here for a long time. I know a lot of things that you don't."

"I'm here all day Sundays, and I haven't seen anything out of the ordinary."

"One full day a week isn't enough, believe me."

"Nevertheless, Molly, talk to the family. It will help you as well as them."

A few days later, Molly told me about her plan.

"I'm asking Mr. Williams for a raise," she said as we walked Bowdie in the park.

"Oh?"

"Yeah. I live far away. I need more money for gas and for the time I spend getting here." She tugged at the leash. "Come on, Bowdie, stop sniffing the grass."

"I don't understand why you don't go directly to Mrs. Bromley. According to you, she's your boss, and she's the one who pays you."

"She thinks I'm overpaid. It's like I have to beg her when I work extra hours."

"But you said she was your boss," I insisted

"She pays me cash with her own money."

"Now, what will you do if he won't give you a raise?" I asked.

"He will."

"Okay, but just suppose he doesn't. What will you do?"

"If he doesn't, I'll quit. It's as simple as that."

"Well, I hope you know what you're doing."

"You should ask for more money too," she suggested. "They think they pay a lot, but that's not so. Mrs. Bromley drains us. We deserve more."

I thought Molly was asking for too much, but after all, what did I know? This was the first job I had ever had.

I was relaxing in the living room when the phone rang. "Lolita, I am Carmen. My husband wants me to talk to you."

Though I had never met Carmen, Mr. William's wife, in person, we had talked a few times on the phone. Although she was from Cuba, she spoke both, Spanish and English fluently.

"Gary thinks we would understand each other better if we spoke Spanish. Can we talk now?"

"Yes."

"Where's Mrs. Bromley?" she asked.

"She's in her room," I answered, curious as what she wanted to talk to me about.

"Can she hear you?"

"No," I said. "I'll move to another room where she can't hear us."

"Good. Gary wants to know if you'd be interested in working full time. Molly's leaving, and we need to know if we should look for a replacement."

Was Molly leaving, or was she being fired? Did I really want to work day and night? Dollar signs danced before my eyes, as well as Mrs. Bromley's angry face.

"Lolita, you don't have to make a decision right now. If you like, think about it tonight and call us tomorrow."

"I'm sorry, Carmen, I'm thinking about it. How much would I get?"

"One hundred fifty dollars a day."

"Can I have some time off in the afternoons?"

"You can have some free time while she naps."

"How about a day off?"

"Jane can watch her one day a week, plus some other times for emergencies. What do you say? I need to know as soon as possible."

"I think it's okay. Yes. Only one thing. I need Wednesdays off, because I teach Spanish that day."

"No problem. Take Wednesday off. Jane can stay with her." She paused. "Is there anything more you want to discuss?"

"When would I have to start?"

"Tomorrow."

"That soon? When is Molly leaving?"

"Gary's going to talk to her tonight. He doesn't want her there tomorrow."

Later that night, I had mixed feelings. It would be nice to make enough money to pay my debts, but what about my friendship with Molly? Maybe if I refused the job, Mr. Williams would be forced to give her the raise she wanted. But on the other hand, we had never been close friends, even if we got along well and I liked her a lot. *My goodness, I should have checked with her before accepting. But Carmen didn't give me time to think.*

Morning found me with unresolved, mixed emotions; I was still not sure I had done the right thing. I concluded that I should have talked to Molly first.

11

Taking Over

Although I hadn't sought this, it troubled me that Molly was gone and that I would profit from it.

I had learned to drive a few years after moving to the United States, and I looked for any chance to drive. Taking Mrs. Bromley where she needed to go was the perfect opportunity to drive. Accustomed to being chauffeured around, driving gave me independence. Behind the wheel, I felt as if the world belonged to me, albeit aware of the responsibility that came along with it.

I wondered how it would be to live with Mrs. Bromley twenty-four hours a day. What if in my joy, I found my sorrow?

I was rinsing out a few dishes when Jane walked into the kitchen.

"Good morning, Lolita," she said, smiling. "My son said you agreed to work full time."

"Yes. I'm glad he asked."

She poured a glass of juice and took a sip. "If you need anything, be sure and call me." She glanced at the door. "I don't want to fire Molly in front of Mrs. Bromley, so I'll explain it to her later."

"Did Mr. Williams talk to her already?"

"No. He left several messages on her machine last night, and she hasn't called back."

"Are you sure she got the messages?"

"Yes, Lolita, I'm sure she did. It isn't the first time she has ignored our calls."

I wanted to ask why she didn't give Molly more notice but decided against it.

"Stay with Betty while I go outside to keep Molly from coming inside," Jane said as she walked away.

I felt badly when I thought about how Molly was going to feel when Jane fired her. Within fifteen minutes, Jane was back.

"Molly is history," she sighed. "She wanted to say good-bye to Betty, but I thought better of it. By the way, Betty likes to eat lunch at Aunt Nelly's. It's on

Gulf Boulevard, right next to Days Inn. They pamper her there, and she loves the attention."

Around noon, Mrs. Bromley knocked at my bathroom door. "Molly, I'm ready for lunch, so hurry up. I am ready." She repeated it many times.

"Please, give me a few minutes."

"What did you say?" she shouted.

I repeated it several times, to no avail, so I opened the door. "Will you please give me a few minutes?"

"Don't you dare shout at me! Hurry up and get ready. I don't like to wait for anyone. I am ready to go, I am ready to go," she chanted. "Why does she make me wait for so long when I am ready to go?" She walked away.

Jane had been right. As soon as we arrived at Aunt Nelly's, two waitresses rushed over to seat us at a table that was reserved for Mrs. Bromley, sporting her name in big letters. The younger waitress immediately brought her a glass of red wine and handed me a menu.

"Is Molly off today?" the waitress asked me.

"Yes," I lied. "She'll be off this week."

"Oh, she didn't tell me," she said. "May I bring you a glass of wine?"

"No, thank you. I'd like coffee."

I looked at the menu and wondered what I could eat. Pasta…everything on the menu included pasta. *If I eat here every day*, I thought, *I'll blow up like a balloon*.

"Are you ready to order?" the waitress asked, placing a basket of hot garlic bread on the table.

"Do you have anything that doesn't include pasta?" I asked.

"We have eggplant prepared any way you like it."

"Do you have grilled chicken or fish?"

"Sorry, no, but we have a tuna platter." She smiled. "That and eggplant are about the only things without pasta."

Mrs. Bromley frowned. "Is Molly being difficult?"

"She forgets that my name is Lolita," I explained. "The tuna will be fine, thank you."

The smell of the garlic bread tempted me. I reached for a piece but pulled my hand back when Mrs. Bromley tapped the table with her knife.

"No bread! You'll spoil your appetite."

"I just can't resist crispy garlic bread," I said, grabbing a slice of toast in spite of her warning.

"Where is your willpower? Don't eat any more," she ordered.

I kept eating.

"Take this away!" Mrs. Bromley yelled to the waitress as she pushed the basket away from me. "Molly is making a pig of herself, and she is too fat as it is."

"Do you really want me to take—?"

"You have no business asking her," Mrs. Bromley snapped. "Take the bloody bread away. I'm the one paying the bill."

The waitress glanced at me, as if asking what to do. I could tell she was embarrassed for me. I didn't want to make a scene.

I winked. "She's really doing me a favor," I said. "I don't need to put on anymore weight…please, take it away."

The waitress picked up the basket and walked away.

"I don't appreciate your incompetent service, so don't expect a tip today!" Mrs. Bromley yelled after her.

"Why are you punishing her because I ate the bread?"

"Because you are too fat and she should have known."

12

Church Morality?

Spring arrived, and with it came its splendor.

As Mrs. Bromley napped, I enjoyed a siesta. I lay down on a chaise lounge and contemplated nature as I watched dozens of seagulls swoop down and eat from a bird feeder. I was grateful for life.

"I will not tolerate this behavior in my house!" Mrs. Bromley screamed coming up behind me. "You are disgusting. Pure pornography! Look at you! Only a cheap prostitute would show her flesh like that." She rushed over and tugged at my shorts. "Cover up your fat legs and ass. What would my grandson say if he walked in right now? Or maybe that is precisely what you want—maybe you want to excite him!"

I jumped to my feet. I couldn't believe what she was saying.

"What are you talking about, Mrs. Bromley. What's wrong with you?"

"Nothing is wrong with me, but there certainly is a plenty wrong with you. This is a decent, moral home and I do not need a provocative, loose woman like you giving a bad name to my home. You are no better than a prostitute!"

"Watch your evil damned tongue!" I shouted. "What the hell is the matter with you? I try to be patient, but you make it impossible. I won't take your insults anymore." I struggled against the urge to slap her face and strangle her on the spot. "You have no right to talk to me like that."

Her hand swung at my face, but I moved just in time to avoid the blow.

"And who said so?" she snapped, glaring at me. "This is my house, and I have the right to do as I darn well please."

I felt my blood rise to my face. I needed to get far away from this bitch or I would explode. I bolted outside and headed down the street in an effort to get rid of the hatred in my heart. I didn't care if she dropped dead while I was gone, and for a moment I wished she would do just that.

It frightened me that my head didn't stop spinning and that just moments before I was angry enough to hurt an old woman. I realized with horror how susceptible to violence humans could be. I walked to the nearby beach in search of solace, which only the ocean could bring. I sat on a bench, concentrated on the blue sky and white clouds, and listened to the sound of the ocean. Slowly, I felt better. Mauricio came to mind: the abuse, the insults, and the humiliation. These two people had so much in common that it sickened me.

I remembered the times Mauricio had accused me of sleeping around. Although I had been extremely patient with him, I could not forget the insults to my integrity. Just like with Mrs. Bromley.

This particular day in Mexico came to mind. I was sitting in the garden, sketching and doodling in a piece of paper, when the maid came rushing in.

"*Señora*," she said nervously, "I'm afraid. I don't know what's wrong, but *Señor* Rimblas just came running into the house. He pushed me and ran upstairs. He had a terrible look on his face."

I ran to the bedroom and flung the door open. Mauricio had emptied my purse on the bed and stood hunched over it, scanning its contents.

"Mauricio!" I screamed. "What are you looking for?"

He poked his index finger in my chest, his face crimson with anger. "Who are you screwing? I should goddamn kill you right now…you whore!"

I leaped at him and raked my nails down his cheeks. He hurled me on the bed and grabbed my neck. I gasped for air. He finally let go, when he realized I had gone limp. I lay there dazed and incredulous.

At the time I was so hurt that I never wanted to see him again, instead, with time, I forgave him. Nevertheless, I could not tolerate any more injustices and insults, specially any affront to my morale, not ever again!

The sea and the rolling of the waves relaxed me, and I was able to see Mrs. Bromley in a different light. I was grateful for my health, so I needed to be sympathetic to someone who was ill, as a way of saying, *thank God for my wellness*. I felt the hatred quenched by mercy, and thoughts of revenge gave way to forgiveness.

"Where have you been?" Mrs. Bromley demanded as I walked back into the house. "I looked all over for you. Why did you disappear leaving me alone, when your obligation is to be with me?"

"I went for a walk."

"Without telling me? That is unheard of."

"I wanted to be alone. I needed to think."

"And what do you have to think about?"

"Come with me. I want to show you something." I took her hand, but she pulled it free.

"Come into the living room with me, please." I stood in front of the nude marble statue. "Do you see that? That is you, and you are naked."

"I was twenty then," she said, with her nose in the air.

"Really?"

"Yes, and I'll be damned if I have the same measurements today."

"Not only are you naked," I insisted, "but your arms are flung up in the air—not a bit of modesty. At least you could have covered your face or your bosom or your…You posed about seventy years ago, when a decent woman would never dare show her ankles. And look there, over the piano. Do you see all those photos of you and your sister dancing on the French Riviera? Both of you are almost naked. Look at your breasts and your legs. Did they call you a prostitute or a whore then?"

"Of course not," she said indignantly. "You should think twice Molly or Lopeta or whoever the bloody hell you are before talking to me that way."

"Teach me; I want to learn. Back then, what did they call women like you who danced almost naked and posed nude?"

"You can be so ignorant! They called it high-class art."

"Then why, in God's name, did you call me a whore and a prostitute just because I was wearing shorts now in the twenty century?"

As though she were Sarah Bernhardt, she waved her hands in the air and paraded around the room. "Poor little Lolita," she informed. "You are suffering from delirium. I really pity you—you and your string of meaningless words. I, on the contrary, relish my past. The European aristocracy fought for the pleasure of meeting me." She walked to the doorway and turned to face me. "And now, Molly—I mean, your majesty Lolita—all you want to do is smear my name. Instead of putting your foot in your mouth, you'd better keep your big mouth shut and study a little bit about art. Now, to put an end to this nonsense, I am going to my room. I do not wish to be disturbed."

I was speechless. Before she left I looked deep into her eyes, trying to understand her complex mind. She had remembered my name, even with an attached ironic tag. *Well,* I thought, *there is a lot more to learn about you Mrs. Bromley.* Unfortunately, I kept forgetting about her decline and my good intentions; compassion and mercy were giving way to murderous rage once more. I took a relaxing breath and figured she must have been manipulative and self-centered all her life, and those traits had only worsened with the illness.

Late that night, I felt the urge to talk to my sister.

"Alma," I said. "I need to get something off my chest."

"Mrs. Bromley again?" she asked.

"Who else? Do you know what she called me today?"

Alma laughed. "Slob, fat, pig, stupid, ignorant—am I right?"

"No, don't be a smart-aleck. She called me a prostitute. Well, actually, she called me a whore. Then she said other terrible things about me. She even said I had fat legs and a fat ass."

Alma laughed again. "Well, there's some truth to that. They are a little...plump."

"Oh, Alma, stop it! I don't know what I'm going to do."

"Then quit."

"You know I can't do that...and why."

"Then quit whining, Lolita. She's the one who has a problem, not you. She's the one that can't change, so if you choose to stay, you must change."

"But I'm trying."

"Then stop trying and just accept the fact that she will only get worse. Calling you a whore is just the beginning."

I knew Alma was right. I must stop complaining. I had to remind myself it was her fried brain talking. *Ay Dios mio, there I go again, forgive me for being impatient.*

The next morning, Mrs. Bromley appeared at my door for the fifth time. "Good morning," she said. "What day is today?"

"Sunday."

"Is it the day to go to church"?

"Bravo Mrs. Bromley. Yes, it is."

"At what time are you going to church?"

Enticed by the idea that I might be able to go to church, I eagerly replied, "Well, I can leave now and just say hello to God and be back in a wink." Then I thought that maybe I could cajole her into going with me. "Would you consider coming with me?"

"At what time do you want to leave?" she asked.

"On Sundays, there are many masses, so as soon as you are ready," I said, thinking that was what she wanted to hear.

"That is the wrong answer. I want to know the exact time."

"We'll leave as soon as you want."

"I said, at what time?"

"How about in forty-five minutes?"

"At what time!"

"Well...10:45," I said, glancing at my watch.

"Finally a correct answer. Now I know when I should be ready."

In fifteen minutes, she was back at my door. "I am ready. I am waiting. I am ready."

"It's too early. We still have a half hour, so let's wait."

"I am ready, and we will leave now. I am ready."

There was no use arguing. "Let's go, then," I said.

"Wait! First be an angel and find my gloves and my hat."

I smiled. "Remember, you don't have gloves or hats. You don't need them in Florida."

"You are a great help. My family should be punished for stealing my gloves. Did I ever tell you they are always stealing from me? I am placing a curse on them not to enjoy a good life, and another on you, for contradicting me." Bowdie jumped at her feet, and she bent over to kiss her. "Oh, my treasure, I know you want to come with us, but you must stay at home. Unfair rules don't allow you in church." She kissed the dog. "Darling, I have nothing for you, except my love...Lolita hides everything from us, even the food. A stranger comes and takes over. Such is the fate of the elderly."

I drove around to kill time. While we were stopped at a red light, she poked my arm and said, "Go on—all the cars are passing us and you are doing nothing, just sitting here. Go! Go on, move! You don't listen. But why are you going to listen, when you know it all?"

I could have explained that we were turning left and the cars passing us were going straight ahead, but I didn't feel like repeating the same thing so she could understand, so I kept quiet.

"Lolita!" she shouted. "I am talking to you! The least you can do is answer me."

"Now we can go," I said patiently. "The arrow is green, and we go left."

"Why did you not say we were going left in the first place? You allowed me to ramble on like a madwoman for your own enjoyment."

"I'm sorry. I should have said something," I said, truly feeling badly.

I drove around some more, and we arrived at St. John's Church close to eleven. I helped her out of the car and started up the steps. An elderly usher rushed to help, taking Mrs. Bromley gently by the arm. She jerked back and shoved him away.

"I'm sorry if I startled you," he apologized.

Her expression changed, and she smiled at him flirtatiously. "Would you please be kind enough to take my arm and guide me?"

He escorted Mrs. Bromley to her seat. She beamed, and to my delight, she behaved marvelously during mass. When it was time for offering peace to one another, the same usher returned and shook her hand.

"Peace be with you," he said.

She smiled and held his hand longer than necessary. "You are very charming, thank you," she smiled, showing her even teeth.

When mass was over, she leaned toward me and whispered, "Let us wait until everybody leaves, to avoid the crowd."

"No problem."

The crowd cleared up and we exited the church. Once out, she asked, "Did you notice the couple in front of me?"

"No, why?"

"I do not believe you. It was very obvious."

"What was obvious?" I asked as I helped her into the car.

"Do not tell me you did not see what they did. It was quite shocking."

"Hmm…" I said.

"No one could have missed such a spectacle," she went on. "They went about their business in plain daylight with no regard to God's presence."

"I was praying and paying attention to mass," I said.

"Do not tell me you were praying with those two exhibitionists in front of you."

I ignored her, wishing she'd shut up. No such luck.

"They were a fraction of a second from having intercourse right there," she continued, snapping her fingers.

I wondered if the usher's closeness had turned her on and she was having delusions. The couple in front of us had only held hands. I was grateful that she had kept her observations to herself during the service.

"They were carrying on and holding hands, looking into each other's eyes, brushing against each other. It was just improper and ghastly. I prayed that God would hold my tongue because I was going to expose them in front of everybody. They should not have left bed this morning if they had not finished their business."

"Please, Mrs. Bromley, leave those two alone. There's nothing wrong with young people in love searching for God. Bear in mind that it's not our business."

She swung around and pointed a finger at me. "That is what you think…but you are wrong. Obscene behavior is every decent person's business. And it is also my business what that old usher did. He approached me again and had the nerve to shake my hand. 'Peace be with you,' he said, but I saw lust in his eyes. He could not fool me. I still recognize lust when I see it. I still remember."

13

Hurricane

Mrs. Bromley sat fixed in front of the TV as it blasted hurricane warnings. "This is a serious matter, Lolita," she said. "Sit here and take note of everything he says. Take control of the situation. We could be out of electricity, water, and food in no time."

"We're north. The warning is for south Florida, far away from here."

"Lolita, you are not being very smart. It is Florida they are talking about, so we are in danger."

"They'll tell us ahead of time if we are in any danger."

"I do not wish to take any risks. I don't want to wait until the last moment." she insisted.

"Don't worry; I've taken care of everything. Nothing will happen," I said, losing count of how many times I had told her the same thing since the hurricane warnings began.

"How do you know? Look at the news. There's panic, pandemonium. They're telling us what to do. Pay attention! Write down where to go in case we have to evacuate."

"I promise I will if the time comes, but now—"

"By then it will be too late," she interrupted. "Are you sure it is blood that runs through your veins?" With amazing agility, she jumped to her feet. "Take me to the store at once!" She went to her bedroom, and came back with her face freshly made up and her hair neatly combed.

"You look elegant and very pretty," I said.

She smiled graciously. "I do look good in blue, but let's not waste time. There is a hurricane on its way."

I sighed. *If you can't win, join in*, I thought. "I'm at your command, my general. Let's go."

"We need candles, water, canned food, a pair of torches, and a lot of matches,"

"You have six torches," I said, hoping to prevent needless expense. "You don't need any more."

"I beg your pardon! Don't you tell me what I need! I know what I need, and most importantly we need plenty of dog food, of course. Oh, Lolita," she said sadly, "if the worst comes, tell the rescuers to forget about us and just save my dearest, faithful Bowdie. I owe her for what she did in Paris." She waved a finger in my face. "Did you hear me, Molly? Am I clear? Bowdie first! I want to save her life as she saved mine."

I struggled to keep a straight face. "Yes, Mrs. Bromley," I replied, "Bowdie first. But please, will you keep in mind that I'm not Molly? I am Lolita."

"*Mon Dieu*, you are concerned with rubbish when we all might perish. It doesn't matter what your name is—Molly or Lolita, or Ginger...you will be just as dead."

I burst into laughter. "You're so right, Mrs. Bromley. We might be wiped off the face of the earth at any time, and here I am, worrying about mundane matters."

"I do not know what is so amusing to you. I don't see anything funny. To the contrary, I foresee a tragedy."

By the time we arrived at the supermarket, she was still obsessing about the hurricane.

"Molly, ask those people around us if they know what is coming our way," she said as we pushed the cart.

"That's very nice of you to think of others, but I'm sure they know."

"I am not so sure, but if they perish, it will be your fault for not telling them. Hurry, take me to the dog section."

As we walked through the pet aisle, she took cans of food from the shelves and tossed them in the cart. "Do not waste time! Help me with my baby's food."

"That's not the kind of food Bowdie eats. We have to see the labels," I said.

"In a life-or-death situation like this, my baby can eat anything to stay alive."

Sometimes I had been able to keep her quiet by saying that she bothered everybody around her with her loud voice. Today it didn't work and her raucous voice boomed throughout the store.

I was aghast when an elderly, distinguished man approached her.

"Julia Child, what a pleasure to meet you," he said.

"Julia who?" she asked.

"Oh, I'm sorry; I thought you were Julia Child. I heard your voice, and...well, never mind. You look like a reigning queen surrounded by her subjects." He said in a French accent.

"*Pardon, monsieur, je ne comprend pas,*" she responded.

"*Vous parley Français*! Ooh la la!" He grinned as he moved closer against the wall to let people pass.

I stood close to them while they spoke in French for several minutes.

She addressed me. "Molly, do you have any of my calling cards with you?"

"Sorry, I don't," I said, withholding the truth. I did so because I didn't want to hand them out to strangers.

"You should carry some of them at all times." She deliberated for a moment. "Well, then please give this gentleman my phone number."

I wrote a made-up number on a piece of paper and handed it to him.

"Will you please write down her name?" he asked.

I wrote Elizabeth and made up a last name.

He looked at the paper, bowed, and kissed her hand. "Elizabeth. You even have a regal name." He kissed her hand. "*Au revoir, madame.*" He released her hand slowly and said, "I'll call you soon."

Mrs. Bromley was beaming when we left the store. "Lolita, can you believe it? I just got picked up. Now we have to find a man for you."

"Oh, no, no, Mrs. Bromley. I'm not interested in meeting a man."

"Why not? Are you a lesbian?"

"No. I'm not."

"Well, I want to double-date, and this Frenchman better have lots of money. I am not paying his way."

"Good," I said, and added, "You don't need anyone taking your money."

"But if he is good in bed, I might pay him. You do not take money with you when you die, you know, and the pleasures you experience in life are, indeed, priceless. I hope he calls me right away. I am getting old, you know. I do not have time to waste."

Driving back to the house with a car full of things that we had no use for, I was sure of one thing: with Mrs. Elizabeth Bromley there was never a dull moment. There were disastrous times, frustrating times, and outrageous times, but boring…not a single one.

For a while, the excitement of meeting the Frenchman occupied all her attention and she kept talking about her date. All of a sudden, the joy vanished lost in the back of her mind, probably forever. Treacherous Alzheimer's was slowly marching on.

I dreaded weekdays because it meant eating at Aunt Nelly's, the Italian restaurant where the menu was all pasta. I would sit there thinking it was a waste of time and money. We ordered lunch, but I only ate the salad. Mrs. Bromley asked for a piggy-bag as soon as she placed her order. The waitress brought her lunch; then, as customary, she put her food into the Styrofoam box without even tasting it. Later at home, it always ended up in the trash. In Cuba, I remembered my mother looking for needy people so she could give them our leftovers. When I had lived in Mexico, I never threw food away, or anything, for that matter. There was always someone in need. Consequently, every time Mrs. Bromley threw away good food, I felt as though I was committing a sin, given the famine in many parts of the world.

At the restaurant, she was irritated because a busboy took her empty plate away.

"You!" she shouted. "Come back here!"

The busboy stopped and looked around.

She motioned him to come to the table. "Yes, you. Do you know what you just did?"

"Ma'am?" he asked.

"Why did you take away my dish?"

"Sorry, ma'am," he apologized. "Your plate was empty."

"Don't you know the rules? You should wait until the knife and fork are crossed, and not until then do you remove the service."

"I'm mighty sorry, ma'am. It won't happen again."

"I'm a very civilized person. If it were some other customer, the manager would have been here already."

"I'm sorry."

She waved her hands. "Go. Go on now. No tip for you."

I decided to take advantage of the situation. Since I didn't like the restaurant this incident would be a good reason not to come back here. Even though I felt sorry for the busboy, I would use him as an excuse to stay away from the Italian restaurant.

We left, and as soon as I started the car, I began my plan. "It was rude of that young man to take your utensils away without even asking you first." I felt shame for the ruse that I was using to keep Mrs. Bromley away from the restaurant, but I justified myself, by thinking that the end justifies the means.

"What young man?" she asked.

"The busboy—he just grabbed your dish away without any courtesy."

I glanced at her; she was where I wanted her to be. I went on, "Besides, he didn't look clean." I racked my brains for more convincing arguments, but I didn't want to slander too much.

"Oh, yes. Although he was black, I recall being very nice to him. I even gave him a generous tip."

Although she hadn't tipped him, I kept quiet about it and went on with my plan. "That restaurant is getting worse by the day. I didn't touch my food, and I saw you struggling to even taste yours."

"That is right."

"We need a balanced diet. Pasta is fattening."

"What do you suggest?"

How nice, I thought, *she's coming around*. "Well, we can try fish. Besides being low in calories, the iodine in fish is good for your brain and will help with your memory."

"Wonderful! That's what I need. I don't know why, but lately my memory is failing me, so you'd better write it down."

"What do you want me to write down?"

"Changing the restaurant. The fish and the memory thing. Write a note and I will keep it in my purse; otherwise, I will forget. Unfortunately, sometimes I do not know where I am, and I can't recall things; when I try, I feel a knot in my head. Hollow, like having nothing inside.

She looked so sad and confused that my heart ached for her.

"What do you think is happening to me?" she went on. "Where have my brains gone?"

"Oh, don't be concerned Mrs. Bromley, I forget things too. And, do you remember *Jeopardy*—you always get the answers, so there's nothing to worry about. We'll eat seafood every day, and I'll give you more ginkgo biloba."

"What's ginkgo? Is that a little lizard?"

"No, you're thinking of a gecko. Ginko is a natural supplement for the brain. It helps circulation."

"Is it obvious, Lolita? Do people notice that I am forgetful?"

"There's nothing to worry about, Mrs. Bromley. You'll be fine. I'll be nearby for whenever you need to remember something."

14

Bryan

"Where are you taking me for lunch?" Mrs. Bromley asked as we drove down Gulf Boulevard.

"Leverocks. Remember? We eat there on Sundays."

"You're mistaken. I have never been in Leverocks."

"You will remember when we get there. It's by the ocean, and the smell of fresh seafood is good for the appetite. We liked the food there."

"You must be hallucinating."

"Wait and see."

We arrived at the restaurant, and the hostess ushered us to a table by the window. I loved looking at the different boats pulled up along the dock. I pointed out the Bay Bridge that divided Saint Pete Beach and the city of Saint Petersburg. We had been there only moments when a young waiter approached us. Before he could speak, Mrs. Bromley asked him, "What is your name young man?"

"Bryan, ma'am," he said.

"Bryan, with that gorgeous smile of yours, you've made my day."

"It comes easily with someone as pleasant and lovely as you."

"*Mon Dieu. C'est formidable.* Bryan, it hurts to pay a bill brought by someone with a sour face. I'd like scotch on the rocks, if you will."

"Yes. Anything for you?" he asked looking at me.

"A glass of Chablis, please."

After a moment, he was back with our drinks.

"Young man, how many children do you have?"

"None."

"Then your wife has you all to herself. I'm sure she appreciates not having anyone to share her handsome husband with. Am I right?"

"Thank you, but I'm not married."

"Poor soul. Do you live by yourself?"

He looked surprised. "If you'll excuse me, ma'am—I'll be right back."

"Lolita, what do you think of him? He's single, and I only questioned him on your behalf. Now we know that he's available."

"Please, don't question him any more. Yes, he seems to be a nice person, but I could be his mother."

"You sure are a cold potato. You're calling him a nice person, when he's adorable, delightful." She licked her lips. "He has desirable lips, don't you think? And he's so cute, so charismatic." She paused for a moment and frowned. "But you know, it is written all over him…I think he is gay. Do you think so?"

"No, I don't, and it's really none of our business."

"You are such a bore! If we don't talk about people we like, what are we going to talk about? Answer me. You sit there like a mummy."

"Talk about him, but don't stick your nose in his business."

"I like him for you. What a pity it would be if he were homosexual, don't you think? It's your loss. Call, what's-his-name?"

"I don't know. Wait until he comes back."

"Bill, my best friend, is a homosexual, you know. Robert trusted him with me and sent us away on cruises when his business kept him at home. Bill understood me like nobody else. I bought him a house and a car; that shows how close we were."

I assumed she was talking about the Bill Straton that she'd had me call many times. For some reasons he was avoiding her.

"Why hasn't Bill returned my calls, Molly? You did leave messages, did you? Something must be wrong. Do you think we should go to Cocoaa Beach and find out?" Before I could answer, she swung around and called out to a passing waiter, "Where's…what's-his-face? I just found him, and he disappeared. Be an angel and get him, will you?"

"Yes, ma'am. I'll get Bryan," the waiter replied.

Several minutes passed, and I could see that Mrs. Bromley was anxious, as she kept looking around the room and asking anyone who walked by where Bryan was. When she saw him approaching our table, her face brightened.

"Yes, ma'am," he said. "What can I do for you?"

"We come here often on Sundays, but I haven't seen you before," she said.

"Sometimes I work private parties on weekends."

"It figures," Mrs. Bromley said. Then, to my embarrassment, she asked, "Do you live alone or you have a partner?"

"With my dog."

"Bravo," she said, shaking hands with him. "I knew there was something very special about you. Tell me everything about your adorable dog."

"My pride and joy is a Pekinese. I'm crazy about her."

"Oh, too bad it's not a male. We could be celebrating a wedding between them and have grandchildren. My treasure's also a female. Bowdie's her name."

"My dog's name is Diamond," he volunteered.

"Good. I'm sure she's a jewel. No pun intended."

He produced a picture from his shirt pocket and handed it to Mrs. Bromley.

"She is my roommate and my partner. She's everything to me."

Oh, lord, I thought. *Mrs. Bromley has found her soul mate.* They both used the same lingo when referring to their dogs.

"May I keep this photo? My baby will be delighted to meet her new friend."

"Sure. I have plenty."

She placed the picture in her purse. "I'll bring a picture of my Bowdie tomorrow. Will you be here then?"

"Yes, ma'am, I'll be here."

"Now, Bryan, I want to play Cupid with your Diamond and my Bowdie."

He laughed. "Ma'am, they are both females."

"Oh, but you know very well that that doesn't mean they can't be each other's better half. Granted, they won't have babies, but they will love each other just the same."

He frowned. "I beg your pardon?"

"I know what I'm talking about…and so do you."

He kept quite for a moment. Finally he said, "No, ma'am, I'm afraid I don't."

"We all need that special significant other." She smiled coyly. "Even if that significant other is of the same sex, we need a companion. A couple is a couple, and the rest is for you to figure out. You decide how to make it work."

Bryan had a puzzled look on his face. He glanced at Mrs. Bromley and then at me as if to say, *what is going on here?* I didn't have a clue what Mrs. Bromley was implying but I guess Bryan did. After a few seconds he smiled kindly at Mrs. Bromley and asked.

"It's up to us to make it work, huh? You two ladies make it work?"

I looked at both of them in disbelieve. *Are they saying what I think they're saying?* I was dumbfounded. I felt my face flush.

"Mrs. Bromley winked at him and gave him a knowing smile."

Bryan burst out laughing. "Ma'am, I would love to stay and chat, but duty calls. I'm really looking forward to your next visit, but now I have to get back to my other customers."

Despite my embarrassment, I felt good knowing that Mrs. Bromley was having such a wonderful time. It was a blessing when he brought the bill and she didn't object; on the contrary, she was very generous with a large tip.

"This is to buy something for the future bride," she said.

Moments later, she said, "Lolita, don't let me forget—what's his name?"

"Bryan."

"I trust you won't let me forget him, and I want to come back tomorrow. Oh, and remind me to bring the bride's picture. We must arrange their wedding. If you keep talking about him constantly, I will keep him alive."

What a difference in her tone! It goes to show; how often people's actions are guided by how they feel inside. When you are unhappy and empty, you project bitterness, when you are contented you project kindness. Now that Mrs. Bromley was excited and motivated she was generous and pleasant. Usually when we had a large bill, she argued and complained all the way home about the lousy food and poor service. She never left a tip appropriate to the size of the bill. It was always two dollars—that is, if she liked the service.

As soon as we got in the car I asked. "Mrs. Bromley, do you still think that Bryan is gay?

"Bryan? Who is Bryan? Do I know a Bryan?

"Our nice, good-looking waiter. He owns a dog. You told him I was a lesbian. Did you tell him we both were gay?" I shot the questions a mile a minute.

"Are you asking me something? Or are you telling me something? You seem distraught. Are you alright?" Mrs. Bromley spoke in a surprisingly kind voice.

"Mrs. Bromley, I don't like to be called gay. Before you called me a whore, and now you say I am gay? It's an insult. It is embarrassing."

"An insult? What are you talking about Lolita? Why would being gay be an insult?"

"Well…you know…well" I stammered.

"Just what I thought. You have no reason. You may prefer a man or a woman; dogs or cats. Who cares? It is just a matter of choice."

I thought about that a moment. It made sense. I've no reason. As a matter of fact, it made a lot of sense coming from Mrs. Bromley. If she could only be so accepting of blacks, children, and employed older women and so on and so forth, life with her would be so much easier.

For the next couple of weeks we had lunch at Leverocks every day. We would ask the hostess for Bryan, and she would take us to one of his tables. Mrs. Bromley looked radiant after all the attention she received from her new friend. They exchanged new pictures of their dogs, and a special bond developed. For the first time since working for Mrs. Bromley, I enjoyed lunch. She acted delightful and spirited.

I told Mr. Williams and Jane about the good times we were having at Leverocks with a gay waiter. Their negative reaction surprised me.

"Please, Lolita," Jane said, "don't take her there anymore."

"Why not?" I asked, baffled by her attitude.

Mr. Williams laughed. "Lolita, you don't know this, but my grandmother's weakness is homosexuals. She has spent a fortune on her friend Bill and we don't want any more problems. Keep her away from that young man and from that place, please."

"But she's with me. I'll keep things under control."

"That's what you think," Jane said. "She's sneaky enough to find a way to give him her business card, or ask him for his phone number."

"But she hasn't done that," I insisted. "And I won't leave her alone."

"If you go to the bathroom or—"

"Jane," I interrupted, "she's never out of my sight. Believe me."

"Don't think we're being unreasonable," Mr. Williams said. "I know you're doing your best, but it won't work with her. When she wants something, she finds a way to get it, regardless."

I was determined to convince them, so I gave the matter another try. "But she hasn't tried to do anything. Maybe when she was younger, she gave men gifts. She can't retain a phone number now, so she wouldn't call anybody. She lives only the present."

"She's not out of it yet," Jane said. "She still has many moments of lucidity. That's all she needs to get in trouble, Take my word for it."

"She's so happy when she talks to him, and because of that, she's sweet the rest of the day."

"I know you mean well, but I know what I'm talking about. Someday I'll tell you more about her adventures with Bill," Jane said. "I'm sorry, but for now, no more Leverocks. Try to understand my position...our position. We've been taken in the past."

And that seemed to be the end of Mrs. Bromley's interlude with Bryan and Diamond.

Days passed by and we tried other restaurants—even another Leverocks in Madeira Beach—nothing made her happy. One moment she was mean, and the next she was even worse. No matter what restaurant we were at, she'd ask for Bryan, the waiter who owned a Pekingese dog. Then she showed the waiters the dog's photo.

After several weeks, I thought it was safe to go back to Leverocks. I thought that by then she would have forgotten Bryan, because for several days she hadn't inquired about him.

When we got in the restaurant I asked the hostess not to seat us in Bryan's section. Once we were ushered at another server's station, Mrs. Bromley asked, "Where's…what's his-name? You know, the handsome blond with the adorable dog?"

"Tell her you don't know, please," I quickly whispered to the hostess.

"I haven't seen him today," she complied.

"Is he well?"

"Oh, yes. He's well."

"And Diamond?" Mrs. Bromley asked.

It was amazing that she remembered Bryan and even the name of his dog.

The hostess smiled. "Your waitress will be with you shortly."

I studied the menu and selected our favorite shrimp dinners, while Mrs. Bromley kept glancing around. Suddenly, she shouted, "Young man, come here! You, come over here!"

Bryan hurried to our table. "Long time no see. I've missed you."

"I looked for you every day," she said sadly. "Were you sick?"

"No, ma'am, I've been here most of the time."

"Lolita, tell him how we've been looking for him."

I smiled at him and nodded.

He smiled back. "I'm happy to see you again," he said. "Now, would you excuse me? I have to pick up an order."

Mrs. Bromley grabbed his arm. "Wait! You have to serve us."

"I'm sorry. This is not my table, but I'll be back to check on you later."

"Damn it, Molly. What the hell's wrong with him?" She shoved her water glass across the table.

I tried to explain why he couldn't wait on us, but she didn't care to listen.

"This much money for a lousy meal!" she said when the check came. "Make sure not to bring me here anymore."

"Mrs. Bromley, please lower your voice."

"I lower it when I want to. Right now, I want to leave." She got up and headed for the door.

As we approached the front desk, she turned and walked into the hall.

"This isn't the way out," I said, taking her arm.

"Leave me alone. I'm waiting for Bryan."

"Please, let's go," I said, pulling her gently.

"I need to talk to him privately."

"That's fine, but not now, he's busy."

"I'm not moving," she insisted. "I'm waiting right here until I see him!"

I remembered what Jane had said several weeks before: "She'll do anything to get what she wants." At the time, I didn't believed her.

"If you do that, you'll get him in trouble. We'll call him from home later," I said, trusting she'd forget all about it once at home.

"Don't play smart with me. We don't have his phone number."

"But I do. I'll even make the call for you."

"You better; otherwise, I will put a curse on you."

I didn't take her back there anymore, but I burned with curiosity to learn more about her relationships with homosexuals.

At a later date, Jane told me the story about the close and odd relationship between Mrs. Bromley and Bill, the gay friend who escorted her on cruises around the world.

When Mr. Bromley died, Bill took over and managed Mrs. Bromley's fortune and helped himself to quite a bit of it. Jane said that Mr. Williams intervened when his grandmother began showing symptoms of Alzheimer's. They went to court, it was a big scandal and it cost a fortune in lawyers' fees. They were able to get back several original paintings and costly pieces of art from Bill's possession. At the moment some of them were securely locked away in the room upstairs.

15

Leti and Japhlet

I hadn't seen my children for a long time when an unexpected joy came into my life. Leti, my youngest daughter and her sixteen-year-old son Japhlet, came back to Florida to live in my house. She had been living in Mexico since her divorce.

It was difficult for her to understand how I could live in someone else's house as a companion. She eventually understood the need for me to work so I could make the mortgage payments. It also upset her that I was no longer attending my writers' group.

I wanted to introduce my family to Mrs. Bromley, but I was afraid of what she might say because of Japhlet's long hair, earrings, and cut off blue jeans.

Eventually, I took the chance and brought them to meet Mrs. Bromley. To my surprise, she overlooked his appearance and was very sweet to him.

"What's your name, young man?" she asked.

"Japhlet."

"What?"

Japhlet repeated his name several times.

"I never heard that name before. Do people call you anything else?" she asked.

"Well, my middle name is Daniel."

"Ah! *Voila*! I'm going to christen you Danny. Do you like that?"

"That's fine. Call me what you wish."

"So you're Danny's mother?" she asked, turning to my daughter. "What's your name?"

"Leti."

"Leti? It's almost like mine. My name is Betty." She leaned over to Leti and grabbed a bunch of her hair. "It looks as if your head is in flames. Who has red hair in your family?"

"There are many redheads in my father's family. His hair is dark and his mustache is red."

"Oh la la…What a combination." She smiled in a friendly way and asked, "How would you like some tea in the dining room, in our best china?" Without waiting for an answer, she turned to me. "Molly, prepare the tea, will you?"

I was puzzled by her kindness and delighted that she was so gracious to my family. We enjoyed tea in a cordial ambience.

"So, I understand that you're British but lived in France and danced with your sister all over," Leti said, sipping her tea.

"Ah, yes," Mrs. Bromley said, smiling and looking up at the ceiling lost in thought for a moment. "We danced for dukes and princes in Belgium and France and all over Europe. We replaced the Dolly Sisters at the Lido."

The memories clearly brought her immense joy. She went on, "My sister was bosom buddies with the queen! They never slept together you know. No funny business…"

Leti and Japhlet just nodded.

Her insistence on that part of the story, which was repeated every time the past came up, made me quite curious about her sister.

Leti and Japhlet offered to watch Mrs. Bromley on Saturdays so I could go to my writers' meetings. Since writing had been my therapy and a very important part of my life, I was happy and grateful to my daughter for that opportunity. We agreed to start the following week.

When they arrived the following Saturday, I gave Leti a crash course on Alzheimer's and particularly Mrs. Bromley's *version* of it.

I enjoyed the morning with my writers' group. Then I took advantage of my day off and spent it catching up with friends and running errands. Finally, I returned to work, praying that Leti's first day with Mrs. Bromley hadn't been as difficult as mine had been.

I returned in the evening to find my daughter straightening up the kitchen. "Well, *mi amor*," I said, "how did everything go? Any problems?"

I was alarmed when I saw Leti's eyes fill with tears. "*Mamita*, I don't want you working here anymore. As soon as I find a good job as a teacher, you have to quit."

"Honey, that's impossible. Salaries in Florida are very low, and with the ridiculous salary teachers make, we might only have enough to pay the electric bill." I laughed.

"But I'm scared," Leti said nervously. "I want you out of here as soon as possible. I know we'll manage somehow."

"What happened to make you so upset?"

Leti called her son. "Japhlet, please go entertain Mrs. Bromley. Keep her away from *abuelita's* room. We need to talk."

As soon as he left, we went to my bedroom, and Leti closed the door. "Mrs. Bromley hates you," she said, fighting back tears. "I don't want you working for someone that is so mean to you."

"Leti, please, why are you saying such things? She's a sick woman."

"She doesn't want you working for her. She forgot you're my mother and said awful things about you."

"Let her say mass if she wants," I said. "I need to work. I can't leave this job. Besides, Mr. Williams is satisfied with my services, and he trusts me."

"*Mamita*, she's going to talk to him. She wants you out and Japhlet and me to replace you. She offered me anything I wanted, even a new car, and that she would double my salary, no matter what it was. Then she shouted, 'That damned Lolita took over my house and she's cold and mistreats me.'"

Leti put her arms around me. "*Mamita*," she said, "I can't stand for anyone to criticize you that way."

"I know she likes to criticize, but that's the way she is with her family. Maybe she thinks I'm part of the family. Don't pay attention to what she says. You don't understand how her mind works. Alzheimer's is destroying her brain; she is demented."

"No. I don't think she's that sick," Leti insisted. "When she asked for you, I said you were having a day off to rest. She looked at me and screamed, 'That's a lie! Lolita's a liar! She's not resting; she's having an affair with a man.' Then she said she was putting a curse on you. You'd break your back, and she wanted you back here in a stretcher, because that would amuse her. Then she laughed like mad."

I tried not to let my concern show. "We must keep in mind—"

Leti interrupted, "Never mind that. Listen to this. After her nap, she said she had a vision of Japhlet dressed in blue. She wanted to see Danny all dressed up like the Blue Boy from Thomas Gainsborough's painting."

"Who's Danny?"

"Remember when they first met?"

"Oh, yes, she baptized him Danny." I laughed. "Don't you see how sick she is?"

"There's more. She wanted to buy a blue silk outfit for Japhlet, so she wanted to know in what boutique I shop for his clothes. I almost told her consignment shops, but instead I said in any department store. Then she said, 'Okay, let's go to the mall.' I tried to talk her out of it, but she insisted on going."

I couldn't believe what I was hearing. "Leti, you didn't take her to the store, did you?"

"Yes, I did. We drove to the mall, and I rented a wheelchair. We strolled to one of the big stores and walked through the boys' section, looking for the perfect blue shirt. Finally, she found one. When Japhlet started rolling his eyes, I assured him that he didn't have to wear the shirt and we could later give it to someone in need.

She held the shirt up like it was some kind of trophy. Then she wanted Japhlet to try on short pants. Japhlet let out a no way, so she agreed to look for slacks. She spotted some blue jeans and exclaimed, 'Ahh…blue!' Japhlet quickly found his size before she changed her mind."

"What happened then?" I asked, afraid of what I would hear.

"She told the salesman to throw his clothes away because Danny was going to wear the new outfit home."

"Did he?"

"No. I told her I would wash the new clothes first, and she agreed by saying, 'If I have waited this long to see my Blue Boy, I can wait a bit longer.'"

"My love," I said, "I'm so sorry I put you and Japhlet through this."

"I don't mind that. What hurts me is the way she offends you."

"Remember, it depends on who gives offense. She doesn't have the power to offend me; I have become impervious to her insults. They are not painful anymore. Don't be concerned, and remember that I love you."

"But I'd like to know why she's so sweet to me and so mean to you."

"Darling, it's a mystery how her mind works."

"Well, let me finish. You won't believe what she said then."

"Oh, yes, I will believe anything about Mrs. Bromley."

"So, in a theatrical manner, she said to Japhlet, 'Danny, turn into the Blue Boy right now. Wear your new outfit home and throw away your old clothes.'

I convinced Mrs. Bromley that Japhlet would wear the outfit later, after taking a shower. Oh, *Mamita*, it was funny in a way. But then she wanted his hair the same length as the Blue Boy, and again I talked her out of it. When we arrived at the house, I hid the painting, hoping she'd forget about the darn Blue Boy."

"*Mi chiquita*, that was nice of her to buy him clothes. Do you think it was true? You know…about the dream?"

Leti shrugged. "Maybe she just didn't like the way he looked and made the whole thing up."

"She doesn't care about anybody's feelings," I said. "However, I think she was very nice to Japhlet, overlooking his long hair and his earring in spite of her strict, conservative upbringing. You know that she always asks me to change clothes whenever she doesn't approve of them, but she never offers to buy anything."

"She's careful not to insult Japhlet. She asked him when he was going to cut his hair, he said, 'Soon,' and she asked, 'In June?' He said louder, 'Soon!' and she insisted, 'in June?' Oh, Mother, sometime she's so cute."

"I don't know, but the truth is that when she's around, there's never a dull moment.".

"And the good thing is that she really likes Japhlet," Lety said

"That's amazing, because she doesn't like children, and certainly not teenagers."

"Well, Mother, since she likes art so much, I promised to take her to the Museum of Fine Arts next week."

"She'll forget your promise. Don't take her anywhere—it's more than enough to deal with her here."

"I feel good about having her do something else besides shopping. Leave it to me."

The following Saturday I came back from my day off, hoping that Leti had not taken Mrs. Bromley to the museum.

"Oh, yes, *Mamita*, we went," said Leti when I asked.

"Oh heavens, did you risk—?"

Leti interrupted. "It was fun, in spite of all the embarrassment she cost us."

"Leti Bire, you're incorrigible."

"Do you want to know what shamed me the most?" she asked.

I laughed. "I'm afraid to find out."

"I rented a wheelchair and we strolled through the galleries. When she began to talk in a very loud voice, Japhlet told me he would wait outside, and left me alone with her. At every painting we stopped, she asked me to read the name of the artist. If she recognized it, she would praise the painting, but if it were an artist unknown to her, she would say nasty things—"

I cut in. "Oh, no! Like what?"

"Well, things like: What an ugly painting. Do you call it a classic? This is a waste of my time and of my money. His family may know him, but I really don't care. I'm not interested in mediocre art. Go on. People looked at us as if we were weirdoes. So, *Mamita*, I wheeled her out of there as fast as I could."

"I suppose you're never going to take her out again," I said.

"You're wrong. Listen to this. Since she loves animals so much, I'll take her to the Tampa Zoo next Saturday."

"You mean you didn't have enough, with what happened today?"

"Relax, mamita."

When they arrived the following Saturday, I asked Leti if she had plans for the day.

"Oh, yes. We're going to the zoo," she said, as if she were taking Mrs. Bromley around the corner.

"I hoped you were joking last week." Then, a bit worried, I asked, "are you sure you want to drive all the way to Tampa?"

"Why not? I have a map and a full tank of gas."

"You don't have to do that. Take her to a park or to the beach."

"At her age, the poor thing doesn't have much time left to enjoy what she still likes in life. I know she adores animals."

I was proud of Leti's compassion, but after the experiences she had gone through, I feared she was looking for trouble.

"*Chiquita linda*," I said. "Even though she likes paintings, her behavior was deplorable in the museum. I don't understand how you dare take her anywhere again. What about Mr. Williams—?"

"Oh, yes! I told him we were going to the zoo, he laughed and told me to leave her there!"

"That's funny."

"Go say good-bye to her, or she'll complain all day that you left without telling her."

"Oh, yes. She always complain that people leave without saying goodbye." I went to her room. "Mrs. Bromley, I came to say good-bye."

"And where are you going?"

"To my writers' group, but Leti and Japhlet are here. They'll stay with you."

"I pay you, Molly—"

"Mrs. Bromley, good morning," Leti said as she entered the room.

She smiled when she saw Leti. "Now I'll have a really good day."

"I'll see you tonight, Mrs. Bromley. I love you," I said as I walked out of the room.

"Hypocrite!" she yelled.

When I heard what she said, I stood by the door to hear what else she had to say.

"Lolita just said she loved me, and yet she leaves me on a special day like this. If it were not for you—"

"Mrs. Bromley, this is Saturday, the day she goes to her writing group."

"But she should stay with me on this special day."

"Why? What's special about this day?"

"It's Christmas, of course."

I returned that evening, curious to find out how my adventurous daughter fared in her endeavor. To my delight, Mrs. Bromley was already asleep. Japhlet was in the kitchen playing his guitar, and Leti was in my bedroom, watching TV.

"Leti, how did it go? Did you go to the zoo?"

"Of course…and I was really astonished. Mrs. Bromley was absolutely charming this time. You should have seen how sweetly she talked to the animals—especially to a giraffe. She pointed to it and said, 'You're lucky to be so close to heaven. I wish I had your long neck so I could talk to God and show my diamond necklace and have everyone appreciate it.' Then she told the camel, 'Beautiful thing, I know you can spit, but I don't want you to try it on me, so behave.'"

All of a sudden, Mrs. Bromley pushed the door open and addressed Leti, ignoring me. "Leti come, you must hear Danny play the guitar."

I made the motion of following them, but the look of scorn on Mrs. Bromley's face and her attitude stopped me cold.

"Come with us, Mom," said Leti enthusiastically

"I prefer to stay, honey."

"You sure?"

"Positive. Don't worry, I'm happy to stay, there's a lot I need to do." I said

They left, and I put Leti's stuff in her bag. I was relieved to see that Leti and Mrs. Bromley were getting along, despite Leti's qualms.

About half an hour later, Leti returned to my bedroom looking puzzled. "*Mamita*," she said, "after listening to Japhlet playing his guitar, I went to fold the laundry, and I overheard Mrs. Bromley and Japhlet talking. I wanted to laugh, but at the same time, it worried me."

"Oh, lord, what did she say now?"

"Proper Mrs. Bromley asked my sixteen-year-old if he had a girlfriend."

"Well, there's nothing wrong with that."

"Of course not…but hear the rest and I'll try to quote: 'Danny,' she said, 'how far have you gone with a girl?' 'What?' he asked. Then she said, 'Have you ever gone all the way with a woman?' Japhlet chuckled and said, 'Well…' And this so-called old-fashioned lady asked, 'And how about a boy?' Japhlet said quickly, 'Of course not, Mrs. Bromley.' 'Has a man ever proposed anything to you?' 'No!' said Japhlet. She clapped her hands loudly and exclaimed, 'Good! You are a clever boy! Monkey business is risky business. My advice, young man, is that it's better to play with yourself and avoid whores and diseases.'"

16

Boy or Girl?

As time went on, I managed to make large payments on my mortgage and on my credit cards. Leti and Japhlet continued to cover for me on Saturdays, and I was pleased with how smooth things were going.

One Saturday evening I came back from my day off and the sadness on Leti's face concerned me. She threw her arms around my neck and said, "Mrs. Bromley keeps finding fault with you. It seems like she forgets everything, yet she's unmerciful in her criticism and complains about you."

"Honey, ignore her. It's just nonsense."

"I try, but I can't. Today she wished that you would have a stroke; a miserable life empty of love and care; and that you were in a stretcher with broken bones."

I had to laugh, "Baloney, that's typical, she forgets everything faster than an ice cream melts over heat. Ignore her like I do; she's sick and bitter."

"That's no excuse. I don't like the mean vibes she sends you."

"She gets her kicks criticizing others. Don't let her get to you."

"But when she insults you, I want to make her eat her words." Leti kissed me, and went for a glass of water. "Do you want one?"

"No, thanks."

When she came back with the water, she looked puzzled. "My feelings for her confuse me. I don't know why, in spite of it all, I like her. She's witty, and even when she's in a bad mood and cursing, she's amusing. I never met anyone like her."

"Good, *chiquita linda*! Then stay with her on Saturdays and Sundays too."

"Oh, no! Once a week is enough, listening to her repeat the same stuff over and over again."

"Absolutely the way I feel." I patted her head and said, "Did you ask her for help with your French?"

"Oh, yes. It's fun. She loves to have me asking about pronunciation and the like. She encourages me."

"Good, she feels needed. How about Japhlet and his guitar?"

"She keeps telling him, 'What are you playing? I can't hear you.' He keeps answering, 'It's an electric guitar, and it needs an amplifier.' Then she'll say, 'Bring the amplifier next time.' This routine happens often. She usually asks, 'Do you sing? You know, it's very important to be able to accompany your music with your voice.'"

"She never stops amazing me. With her, you never know what tickles her fancy." I said, recalling how hard it was for me to please her.

"No doubt she's happy with us. She asked Japhlet to take care of the dog's medicine." Leti sipped her water and went on. "She talks to the dog as if it were a human. 'Bowdie, my treasure, go with your little friend.' Blah, blah, blah. I'm telling you Mom, she's quite a character. What a pity she spoils everything for me when she talks badly about you."

"So then I'm not imposing on you."

"*Mamita*, I'll do anything to help you," Leti said comfortingly.

Margarita, my seventeen-year-old granddaughter, came from Minnesota for the holidays. The day after Christmas, Leti, Japhlet, and Margarita came to spend some time with me at work. Mrs. Bromley seemed pleased to meet my granddaughter and was in her charming mood. In the midst of a conversation, she looked intensely at Margarita and bluntly asked, "I have a question for you, young…well…how should I address you?" She giggled. "With your hair so short, I can't figure out if you are a girl or a boy."

Margarita was silent for a moment, and then said, "Does my name, Margarita, help you? Or maybe the sound of my voice will give you a hint?"

Mrs. Bromley hesitated before saying, "You never told me your name before. Come on, tell me: are you a boy? You must be, with that short, short hair."

Margarita blushed and coughed nervously. "Mrs. Bromley, I am a girl. F-E-M-A-LE."

"I don't believe you. You must be a boy." She walked up close to my granddaughter and patted her breast. Margarita pulled away abruptly.

"You're right; you are a girl."

Japhlet contained his laughter, then jumped to his feet and walked out of the room, saying, "I'm leaving before she wants to find out if I am a boy."

My friend Irene was moving to another state and her friends organized a farewell party at the exclusive Belleview Biltmore Resort. I couldn't find anyone to stay with Mrs. Bromley, and I wanted to go to the party very badly. Lety volunteered for my grandson, Japhlet, to get out of school at noon, and I reserved another table for the two of them near our table. I thought Mrs. Bromley would love to have lunch with Japhlet at such a nice place. At the same time, I thought Japhlet would enjoy the good food.

"*Abuelita*, I'm happy to help you out," he said when I asked him, "but why don't you just take Mrs. Bromley with you? Why do you need me?"

"By now, I know better."

"What do you mean?" Japhlet asked

"I took her to one of the luncheons once and I'm still regretting my mistake."

"What did she do?"

"Well, I took her to one of the Belleair Beach luncheons. She wore a fabulous outfit from Paris and everyone at my table was fascinated by her. She was charming and witty while she was the center of attention. Once they turned their attention away from her, she began to complain about the food and the service. Then she accused them of poor manners and being rude to her. I was so embarrassed, I left."

"Oh, boy! But aren't you afraid of another scene?"

"Not really. This time you're going to be with her. She likes you, and she'll be happy in your company."

We picked up Japhlet on the way to the resort. When he got in the car, I greeted him with the usual "*Hola, mi amor, como te fue?*" Mrs. Bromley jumped in. "I can't believe this! Do you know it is bad manners to speak another language in front of people? Are you talking about me?"

"Of course not," I quickly replied. "You are so right. I'm very sorry for my rudeness. It won't happen again."

"*Bon...bon,*" she said, smiling.

Once in the restaurant, I explained to Mrs. Bromley that Japhlet would be her companion and I would be nearby with friends. I thought she understood, and I left.

I was enjoying my lunch when Japhlet came over and whispered, "She's getting mad because you're ignoring her. She said that she hopes you get a stiff neck for not turning around to check on us. Now she's drinking another scotch, and she said that when she's finished, she's coming over here to give you a piece of her mind."

I took a deep breath, apologized to my friends, asked for the bill, and left.

Time passed, and Leti found a job as a fourth-grade teacher in a private school. She could still cover for me on Saturday mornings, so I could continue with my writers' group. Almost every Sunday after mass, I took Mrs. Bromley and Bowdie to my house. My grandson played with the dog, and Mrs. Bromley beamed at the sight of them.

Leti liked her job and loved her pupils, and they developed a wonderful relationship. She sometimes shared with them her experiences with Mrs. Bromley and explained how Alzheimer's was affecting her mind, contributing to her unstable behavior. It got to be a routine: every Monday the pupils asked about her weekend with Mrs. Bromley and Bowdie.

On one of our Sunday visits, Mrs. Bromley was, still more than other Sundays, enthralled watching Japhlet and Bowdie playing with a ball. Leti approached me with the familiar expression that I knew meant she was after something.

"*Mamita*," she said, "will you please bring Mrs. Bromley and Bowdie to my classroom this Friday?"

I couldn't believe she would ask me to do such a thing. "Are you out of your mind? Why on earth do you want to do that?"

"My students want to meet her, that's all."

"Don't you know the kind of chaos she could unleash at your school? To say nothing about jeopardizing your job."

With her voice breaking with laughter, Leti asked, "What does my job have to do with Mrs. Bromley's visit?"

"You can get fired. Do you have permission from the principal?"

"Of course I do. Guest speakers are always welcome. It is good for the children to be exposed to different people and cultures."

"Don't you know how much she dislikes children? In a way, she hates them. Even her own grandson never brings his baby to see her. Doesn't that tell you something? She'll probably make a scene at the school. Remember how she acts in restaurants when there are kids around."

"It would be different in a structured class environment." Leti cocked her head and stroked my hair. "Look at her now. She's happy talking to Japhlet. She's not bothering us, because she's being entertained. Probably the few times she has been around her great-grandson, everyone pays attention to the child, and she can't stand to be ignored."

"That's exactly what worries me…her need to be the prima donna."

"*Mamita*, I'm sure it's going to be fine. The children are very well-behaved, and she will be the center of attention."

I knew that Leti was very persuasive and that no matter what I said, in the end, I was going to give in. Still, I tried again. "What if she yells and is mean to the kids? And what about the dog? Oh, Leti, please don't make me an accomplice to your demise."

"*Ay mami.* How melodramatic! Nothing will discourage me. It will be good for Mrs. Bromley and good for my pupils. They already know a lot about her and her illness." Leti paused, and then added, "I've been preparing them to meet her for a long time now. They know she has Alzheimer's and that she might say something she shouldn't. I instructed them to remain seated and quiet. They'll raise their hands to ask a question and will speak one at a time."

"I still don't see the point of taking an old lady who can't control her reactions, to meet with a bunch of school children. It's unfair to expose your pupils to a deranged woman."

"*Mamita*, don't underestimate Mrs. Bromley. At her age, and in spite of her illness, I'm sure she can still rise to the occasion when it's really needed. I'm very excited about her visit."

"I commend you for that, but I'm afraid…" I tried again, but I knew my words were falling on deaf ears. "I don't want you to go through all the embarrassments that I have been through."

"Embarrassed, me? No way! To the contrary, I'll be proud of her." Leti turned around, placed her arms around my shoulders, and whirled me around. "Oh, Mother, I would like to show today's youngsters that old people might look feeble and act strangely, but in spite of that, they have a lot to offer to the new generation. Each senior citizen carries an encyclopedia of life experiences and knowledge inside their heads. I'm positive that Mrs. Bromley will do a very good job, and mark my words: I have the feelings that we are going to remember this event for time to come."

"Remember what Alzheimer's does to the mind? She can't control her behavior."

"Yes, I know, but I'm going to delve only into her past. We're interested only in her meeting the queen, being attacked in Paris and saved by her little dog, and her dancing days entertaining royalty. I'm sure the children will love meeting such an interesting and extravagant old lady."

"You make it all sound so easy, but I'm worried."

"Relax, *Mamita*. Let Mrs. Bromley enjoy the here and now. She'll relish being in the limelight once more."

"Well," I said, "what if the kids get involved in their own things and ignore her?"

"Stop it. I don't want to hear any more. Just bring my guest of honor and leave the rest to me."

17

Visiting the School

The day to take Mrs. Bromley to be interviewed by Leti's students arrived. I woke up with an uneasy feeling. After freshening up, I went to her room and opened the drapes. Hiding my anxiety, I said cheerfully, "How are you this morning, Mrs. Bromley?"

"Just surviving, that's all." She pulled the sheets up to her chin. "I want to sleep some more. Go away."

"Not today. We're going out this morning."

"What did you say?"

I went closer to her. "Here, Mrs. Bromley, put on your hearing aids, please."

She did and asked, "Why are you here so early?"

"We're going out this morning."

"Do I have a hair appointment?" she asked, brightening up.

Although I wanted to lie and say yes, because she loved to go to the hairdresser, I couldn't. "No, we have to be in Largo soon."

"I don't like people dodging my questions, and I don't like 'soon' as an answer. Give me the exact time and place. Where are we going and at what time?"

"We have an appointment with my daughter Leti at eleven," I said, handing her a silk robe.

"Do I know your daughter?"

I got closer and said, "Of course you do. We spend Sundays with her and Danny, her son."

"Do I like her?"

"Yes. You even said you want her to replace me."

"That doesn't mean anything. I'd like to replace you with anyone."

"What do you have against me, Mrs. Bromley?"

"Number one: you have taken over my house. Number two: my grandson is always on your side."

At last I knew why she resented me. "I'm only trying to run things smoothly in your home, and your grandson appreciates that."

"If that's the case, go to his house and run it for him. This is my home. Now, where did you say we're going?"

"We're going to meet my daughter."

"Do I like her?"

I sighed. "You do. You'll remember when you see her."

"I want to stay in bed some more," she said, tossing her robe on the floor and holding onto the blanket.

I wished my daughter hadn't put me in such a predicament. If Mrs. Bromley wanted to stay in bed, there was nothing that would make her get up.

"You have to get up now if you want to be on time," I said.

"I didn't promise anything to anyone, so I won't move from here." She rolled over on her stomach. "Go away, and don't bother me."

"You promised to meet Leti at eleven today."

"Are you sure?"

"Positive." I went to her closet and chose an outfit that she particularly liked. "Do you want to wear this?"

She turned around and her eyes lit up. "Leave me alone. I'll get ready myself."

When we arrived at the school, I hid my concern and smiled confidentially at Mrs. Bromley.

"I'm going to get Leti, so please wait for us right here. Don't leave the car."

I hurried to Leti's classroom and knocked at the door. She opened it, and I said nervously, "Hurry up. She's outside."

"Calm down, *Mamita*." She turned to her aide. "Miss Burton, please look after the class. Children, I'll be right back with Mrs. Bromley and Bowdie. Remember everything I told you."

As we got to the car, Mrs. Bromley was trying to get out.

Leti smiled sweetly and took her arm. "How are you today, Mrs. Bromley? You look very pretty."

Mrs. Bromley looked at her and grinned. "I remember your smile, young lady."

Leti took charge of Mrs. Bromley, while I grabbed Bowdie. We went into the classroom, which was crowded with excited children. As we entered the children stood and chanted, "Good morning, Mrs. Bromley."

"Oh, la, la! So many children!" she exclaimed.

Leti helped her to an armchair next to her desk. "Mrs. Bromley, would you like to sit here, please?"

"Thank you kindly," she said. "Who's the teacher here?"

"I'm the teacher."

Mrs. Bromley sized her up. "You look like one of your students. You are so petite and frail. Are you able to control your pupils?"

Leti smiled. "I never have problems with them. Thank you for coming to our school, Mrs. Bromley. You have such an interesting life and you have traveled so much; my students want to interview you. Would you be kind enough to answer some questions?"

Mrs. Bromley smiled charmingly. "I'll be delighted."

Leti turned to the class. "Children, have your questions ready. You may begin the interview. One at a time please."

Hands went up in the air. "Oh, dear! That is a lot of little hands," Mrs. Bromley said, with the cutest smile on her face. "You, handsome," she said, pointing to a smiling blonde boy. "What do you want to know?"

The child rose slowly. "Have you ever met a queen?"

"Unfortunately, I never met one, but my sister Zinna was very close to the queen of Spain. They were close buddies. She was free to go in and out of the palace as she pleased. Zinna spoke perfect Spanish."

To my relief she ended it all there. Would I ever understand this woman? How on earth did she have the common sense to select the appropriate words? I hoped she wouldn't say that her sister and the queen hadn't been sleeping together, like she always did. If her mind was so warped, how was she able to circumvent the part of the story unfit for children? My attention went back to the interview.

More hands were waving.

"Oh, la, la," Mrs. Bromley said. "I am impressed. Look at all these little hands! I want to please all of you, lads." She pointed to a thin girl. "What's your name, young lady?"

"Martha."

"Pretty girl, pretty name. What's your question, Martha?"

"What's your favorite food?"

"Well, I love duck *à l'orange*. I can never have enough of it. Now you, towhead."

"Do you like gravy?" he asked. "Miss Leti said you did."

She burst into laugher. "Oh, yes, lots of it. I like mashed potatoes swimming in gravy." She signaled to an African-American girl.

I looked at the ceiling nervously, afraid of what she might say. I remembered how prejudiced she was.

"What's your question, pretty girl?"

Surprised I thanked God, and from that moment on, I relaxed. For some inexplicable reason, she sounded so normal and controlled that I forgot how mean she could be. No doubt she relished being the center of attention.

"Do you like pets?" another child asked.

"I don't think I could live without them. What do you want to know, young man."

"Has your dog saved you from muggers?" he asked.

She pondered for a moment. "No, I don't think so."

"Mrs. Bromley," Leti interjected. "Do you remember how Bowdie saved your life in Paris when a man attacked you?"

With a vague look, in a soft voice, Mrs. Bromley said, as to herself, "Funny, I don't recall." The smile disappeared, and she pointed to a little girl in the front row. "You are next, young lady," she said sadly, in a little voice.

"Have you ever lived in Paris?"

"Heavens, yes." Her smile returned. "How I miss Paris and my friends. I still have my flat there, close to a plaza full of quaint boutiques." Then she asked another dark-skinned girl, "You, dear. What's your name?"

"Rashni."

"Pretty name. Are you from India?"

"Yes, madam."

"I have good memories of India. And what do you want to know?"

"Do you like flashlights?"

"You mean torches. I can't sleep without a dozen under my pillow." With a twinkle in her eye, she pointed to a boy. "Now you, handsome."

"May I pat Bowdie?"

"Wait for later. Now you, young man."

"Have you ever been to the Eiffel Tower?"

"Yes. I used to bike to it from my flat. Now you, pretty girl—your question."

"Have you visited the Leaning Tower of Pisa?"

"I posed for news photographers in front of it. Now you," she said to another girl.

"Do you like to dance?"

"*Mon Dieu*...and how! I danced on the stage in Paris with my sister Zinna. We took over the Dolly Sisters' show." She rolled her eyes. "Memories...! Maurice Chevalier was a big movie star, but you might not have heard of him. He courted me at that time. He was in the first row nightly with flowers for me. I performed for the cream of the crop. Oh, well…Now you, handsome."

"How old are you?" the boy asked.

"A taboo question, young man. A golden rule: do not ask a lady her age." She smiled impishly and waved a finger at him. "But I'll tell you, because I'm beyond being coquettish. I'm pushing fifty-five. Now you, young man."

I suppressed a laugh. *How can you get rid of so many years at once, Mrs. Bromley? Ten or fifteen might be credible, but…*A boy asked about my grandson, so I paid attention.

"Do you like Miss Leti's son, Japhlet?"

"No. Who's he?"

"He played the guitar for you," the boy said.

"Ah, yes, you mean Danny!"

"Bravo!" I shouted.

It was remarkable that she remembered Japhlet/Danny. The questions went on for a while longer, and when it was time to leave, each child approached Mrs. Bromley, shook her hand, and thanked her for coming.

I was elated with our visit to the school and to see how enthusiastically and kindly Mrs. Bromley responded to the children.

She beamed as we walked away. Halfway to the car, she stopped, placed her hand on my arm, and looked at me thoughtfully.

"You know Lolita, all my life people have pretended to like me, thinking only of what I could give them. Today I was touched by the attention those sweet children gave me without expecting anything in return. They accepted and liked me for who I am. What a fantastic experience! I had a magnificent trip to a different world, where innocent, smiling angels treated me with respect and dignity. Now, listen to me very carefully. What happened here today is something I do not want to forget, but unfortunately we both know I will. It is devastating to know I can't retain anything. I'm holding you responsible to make this memorable day stay with me as long as I live."

Words failed me and I felt tears filling my eyes. It took me a few seconds to regain my voice and my composure.

"Oh, Mrs. Bromley, how do you expect me to do that?" I asked, averting my eyes and tugging at Bowdie's leash.

"Write a detailed note and put it in my purse."

"That's very clever of you. I'll do it as soon as we get to the car." "Every time I open my purse and read it, I'll remember how special those children were." She walked ahead, and then looked around the school grounds. "Why can't I bottle up the wonder of this day and the joy those children have brought me? What's happening to me, Lolita? What's becoming of me? Why can't I remember? Please, I want to know. Get in the car right now and write down everything that happened today before you forget it."

Her sorrowful face filled me with pain. Life could be so cruel. I felt her anguish very close to my heart; I wished I could do something to ease her anxiety.

Although I wanted to cry, I forced myself to smile, and as I fastened her seatbelt and placed Bowdie on her lap, I said gently, "Relax, Mrs. Bromley. Everything's going to be all right. I'll help you to remember. I'll write down everything that happened today."

The fatigue from the hectic day gave way to her familiar confusion. Her moment of lucidity was gone. I thought of the millions of people suffering from Alzheimer's, and to my horror, I realized that I could be one of them someday.

Suddenly, her eyes brightened again, and for a moment, a flash of the wisdom and charm of the woman she had once been returned.

"Lolita, I want you to buy a souvenir for each child. I want them to remember my visit forever."

"That's an excellent idea!" I said. "Do you know what I think would be nice? Let's buy a cake and refreshments and have a farewell party to celebrate their spring vacation."

"No. I want something tangible—a little token for each child, as a reminder of this day and me. I know it will escape my mind soon, but I want them to remember."

"I'll take pictures. Pictures last for a lifetime. We can even provide a magnet, so they can stick the photos on their refrigerators."

She was quiet for a while, seemingly immersed in her thoughts.

"I know what," she said. "I'd like you to buy something the kids can hold in their hands, close to their hearts, and you can still take all the pictures you want."

18

Farewell to the Children

Like Mrs. Bromley, I also wanted to remember those meaningful moments of our visit to the school. I thought it might be better to buy the gifts for the kids while the memories were fresh in her mind. On the way, I stopped at a gift shop and carefully chose twenty little presents.

Mrs. Bromley surveyed my selection on the counter and picked up a doll dressed as a football player.

"What's this for?" she asked. "You aren't going to make me pay for all of these, are you?"

"Remember? You asked me not to let you forget to buy souvenirs for each of the children at the school."

"What children?" she demanded. "I don't like children! Why would I spend my money on them?"

I gently took her hand. "Think hard," I said. "We visited my daughter Leti at her school this morning."

"You're trying to make me crazy," she snapped, pulling her hand away. "You're no help at all. You're losing your mind."

The simple transition of walking from the car to the store had erased the conversation we had just minutes earlier. I felt deep sorrow for her, recalling how badly she wanted to retain those memories.

"Look in your purse, please."

She looked at me defiantly. "Why should I do that?"

"Look inside, please, and then you'll remember."

Fortunately, I had written the note in the car before driving away from school and slipped it into her purse. She took out the piece of paper and read it aloud: "I must remember to buy presents for Leti's pupils. I had such quality time with those children that I want to go back to their school and bring a gift to each one of them, so they will remember our meeting and me forever."

She looked at the note intently. "That's not my handwriting. But never mind, if you say so." She stared into the distance with an empty expression on her face and added, "What a pity...I can't remember a thing, and I feel a knot in my head..." She grabbed her head. "There's nothing in here. My head's empty. I want to remember!"

I flinched realizing her pain. How could I help?

"Don't let it bother you, Mrs. Bromley, I'm sure it will come back to you later."

She looked around and pointed to a shelf on the wall. "I want that little dog. Poor little thing! He looks as lost as I am."

The clerk handed her the stuffed dog, and she kissed it. "Darling, I'll call you Spotty because of your brown spots. Bowdie is waiting for you in the car. Don't get jealous, because I love you both. I promise that neither you nor I will be lonely again."

As soon as we arrived home, I wrapped each toy separately.

Three days later Mrs. Bromley and I delivered the toys to the children. She didn't protest when I explained where we were going, so I assumed it sounded familiar enough for her not to argue about it. As always, I wondered what thoughts lurked in her unstable mind.

The students rose as we entered the classroom. "Good morning, Mrs. Bromley," they chanted. "We're very happy to see you again."

Her face brightened. "Good morning! I am more than happy to see all of you."

I was waiting for her to end the sentence with "happy to see all of you again," which would have been a clue to know if she remembered, but no such luck. I didn't know if she was looking at the kids as if it were for the first time, or if she remembered being here before.

She sat in the armchair, surrounded by the children. "Dear boys and girls," she said, "I brought each of you a memento to take home, so you'll remember me, because unfortunately, I won't."

"Thank you, Mrs. Bromley," the children answered.

"You've given me the greatest gift of my life—you made me feel alive. Looking at you is like returning from a dark tunnel and suddenly seeing the light. Thank you, dears, from the bottom of my heart."

"We made a poster for you," a boy said. Another boy and a girl held up a huge piece of construction paper decorated with red hearts. It read: *WELCOME BACK MRS. BROMLEY. WE LIKE YOU A LOT.*

She started to rise but changed her mind and sat back, smoothed her hair and looked in silence at the children one by one. "Thank you all very kindly. I'd love to remember the name of each one of you, but sometimes I don't remember mine."

I marveled at her interaction with the children. I'd give anything to go into her mind and find out what it registered. What was the cause of her apparent relaxed attitude and the spark in her eyes? Did she recall the children? Or was this a brand-new experience, disconnected from the previous one? Nothing indicated that she felt strange in the surroundings. How and where could I find answers?

To me, this was very odd. Was she stepping back into the past, or perhaps ahead, into the future? But, probably it was better for me not to poke into the unknown and enjoy the moment. I'd leave this mystery to science. I wondered if researches knew already why some patients have longer spans of lucidity than others, and why Mrs. Bromley spoke, sometimes, with such clarity of diction and thought, using long well coordinated sentences.

I interrupted Mrs. Bromley's conversation with the pupils and placed the gifts on the desk. "Do you want to hand the presents to the children?"

"Delighted to do that."

Leti helped to move the armchair closer to the desk and Mrs. Bromley picked up the first nicely wrapped gift.

As she passed out the presents, I took one picture after another of the kids. At the end, I took pictures of Leti and Mrs. Bromley with the children and Leti took one of me with the group.

"Miss Leti, can I show Oreo and Cream to Mrs. Bromley?" a little girl asked.

"Yes…but only from far away," Leti replied.

The girl walked to the back of the room and returned with two pet rats and stood by Mrs. Bromley. I thought she would scream. Instead, she stared at the rats with amusement.

"What cute, furry little creatures!" she finally said. "What are they?"

"Pet rats," Leti said, moving closer to her.

"Do you want to pet one?" the girl holding the rats asked. "They're cool and very friendly."

Mrs. Bromley reached out her hand and gently patted the rat. "It doesn't feel cool at all; on the contrary, it feels warm." Then she stared into the rat's eyes and whispered, "You are so cute, little thing, and your eyes tell me you are smart."

A clear, joyful child's voice asked, "Miss Leti, may I show her Sapphire?"

"Dennis we need to ask Mrs. Bromley first. She might not want to see Sapphire." Leti approached Mrs. Bromley and took her hand. "We have a friendly pet snake, a ball python. Would it scare you if we brought it out?"

"Why, certainly not!" Mrs. Bromley exclaimed immediately.

In a flash, Dennis was back, with the snake wrapped around his arm. He unwound it, and Mrs. Bromley ran her hand up and down its long body. "Oh, la, la! It is gorgeous. *Merci beaucoup* for sharing it with me."

"Mrs. Bromley is cool," said the boy. "Miss Leti, can we see her again? Ask her to be my grandma. I don't have one."

"My little Dennis, that's more complicated, but I can ask my Mom to bring her more often."

Impulsively the boy approached Mrs. Bromley with clear intentions to hug her.

"No!" I blurted out. To mind flashed how she stiffened when I hugged her, and how brusquely she pushed me away. "Don't do that."

"Don't do what?" Mrs. Bromley asked firmly.

The boy stood in place, looking at her with wide eyes.

"I think Dennis wants to hug you but my mother thinks you won't like it," Leti said softly, looking steadily into her eyes.

She frowned. "Who is Dennis?"

"Me."

She looked at the boy for a long while with what I thought was scorn. I restrained my impulse to carry the boy away, far from her grasp and her coldness.

She beckoned the boy. "Come closer, sweetie." Her expression softened when she said, "You can hug me."

Shyly, Dennis approached her. She bent to receive his hug. Suddenly, she drew the child into her arms in a tight embrace.

Emotion overcame me and I couldn't talk. I knew the scene I had just witnessed would be with me forever.

When we were ready to leave, the children gave us flowers and a thank you note. The kids wanted to take Mrs. Bromely to the car, so Leti lined them up in pairs and went with us. They all waved good-bye as the car drove away.

"Where are we going now?" A happy and spirited Mrs. Bromley asked as I drove away.

"We are going to lunch and then home."

"It is not necessary to go home," she answered quickly. "I'm ready to go, I have my passport with me. Let's eat at the airport."

"At the airport?" I asked, surprised. "Where will you be going?"

"Not me, us. To Paris, of course." She paused for a moment. "Are your papers in order? Do you have your passport with you?"

"I didn't know we were going anywhere," I said, humoring her. "I didn't bring my passport. But are you sure you want me to go with you?"

She slapped my hand gently. "Of course, silly. I wouldn't think of going anywhere without you."

I smiled, "How come? Sometimes you don't like me. Do you really want me in Paris with you?"

"By all means!" she exclaimed.

"Why do you want me along?"

The expression on her face changed, and she said solemnly, "Because I trust you more than anyone else." She paused for a moment, and spelled the word trust, then asked, "Do you know the meaning of the word?"

"Yes, Mrs. Bromley."

I wondered if I really knew the exact meaning of the word, because its definition didn't match the way Mrs. Bromley mistreated me. Her unexpected change left me more confused than ever.

"Lolita," she said again, "I asked if you know what 'trust' means."

"Well, at least I think I do,"

"It means to confide in, to rely upon. Because I trust you, I am under your care without reservation. You have a great responsibility on your hands, because I rely on you. Do you hear? You are trustworthy."

I patted her arm. "I'm really confused, Mrs. Bromley. Sometimes I feel like you don't trust or even like me. You asked my daughter Leti to move in with you; what's more, you asked your grandson to fire me because you said I took over your house." I didn't dare remind her that she had called me a whore, a thief and worse. That she had accused me of sexually provoking her grandson. I wanted to remind her of all the other nasty things she called me, but I knew better.

She looked thoughtful as she said, "That's my nature. Usually I don't trust anyone, but you've proven to be reliable and a very important part of my life. I consider you my best friend, and you're doing a perfect job with my house."

Emotion overtook me again, and my heart shattered at the thought that Alzheimer's would sap away her new feelings for me and worst yet what was left of her pride and dignity.

"Oh, Mrs. Bromley, thank you for saying that. It makes me feel so very good to know you appreciate me."

And that was the truth. To know that she relied on me changed the situation completely. This knowledge would help me balance her mood swings and frequent nastiness. Now I could bear anything, even if five minutes from now she reverted to her old self...I'll remember her true feelings and love her to pieces.

She opened a small felt purse. "See here, Lolita. We have enough money to go to Paris and have the adventure of our lives."

"But that's not American money."

"Of course not. It's better, silly. It's French francs and English pounds." She smiled. "I have enough here for both of us."

"Thank you so much for inviting me to go with you to Paris, and thank you for letting me know how you feel about me. I'm sure our relationship will change for the better. From now on, I'm not going to be hurt by the way you treat me."

She looked surprised. "*Mon Dieu*, and how do I treat you?"

"Extremely rude and mean."

For a moment she seemed lost in thought, then she said, "Lolita, have you noticed that lately I have become very forgetful?"

"Yes, Mrs. Bromley. I'm very sorry. I wish I could help you remember more."

"Do you think there's hope for me?" Her voice weakened, and her face was devoid of expression. The focus in her eyes slowly trailed away, leaving in its place the usual vacuum I had come to dread and hate. I vowed that from now on, my heart would rule the way I cared for her. I would give this tortured soul the love and care I had given my own sick mother before she passed away.

I pulled up in front of a restaurant and helped Mrs. Bromley out of the car.

"Here we are, Mrs. Bromley."

I went around the car to help her out.

"I'm fine. I don't need help," she replied firmly, walking ahead of me.

The hostess ushered us to a table. Mrs. Bromley asked immediately for a scotch on the rocks. As she sipped the drink, her expression changed, and she was again the lively Mrs. Bromley. Suddenly she began to read aloud the business signs in a building across from us, a routine to which I had become accustomed.

"XXX Mega Center. Toys, magazines, videos...Shhh: don't tell Mama." She looked at me with wide-open eyes. "Lolita what does that mean? And why shouldn't we tell?"

"I don't know," I said, embarrassed.

"What is triple X?" she asked again.

I moved closer to her and whispered in her ear, "When something is rated triple X, it means pornography, I guess."

"What kind of pornography do you guess?" she asked loudly.

"Women and men having sex on film." I ventured.

With a mischievous expression, she replied aloud, "Oh, la, la. I remember all about that. I think Americans call it hanky-panky. Free membership." She looked at me solemnly. "Why don't we take advantage of the free membership?"

"How's your drink?" I asked, trying to divert her thoughts.

"Weak; too much ice," she said. "Look, Lolita, they have lotions and potions. Exotic clothing. Naughty cards. Gag gifts? Gags—what does that mean?"

"I'll be back in a minute, Mrs. Bromley," I said as I stood up.

"Where are you going?"

"To the bathroom."

I was so embarrassed I didn't know what to do. Not wanting to leave her alone, I walked to the ladies' room area and stood there, hoping that she would forget the darn signs. I took my time, but when I returned she was still fascinated with the advertisements. I ignored her questions, but it was hard to ignore her shouting.

"Gags. Mags. What are those?"

"I don't know. It doesn't matter."

"Mags. Toys. Movies. Buy three and get one free. *Mon Dieu*! That's a good deal!"

"Please, Mrs. Bromley, read to yourself," I said, trying not to let my frustration show.

She sipped her drink. "Why? I'm not bothering anyone."

I was relieved when the waiter brought our order. Maybe now she would start eating and be quiet. But no such luck.

"Tourist guides. Lingerie leather. Spice it up…you'll love it! Swinger mags."

She called a young waiter over. "What does 'swinger mags' mean?"

"I'm not sure," he said. "I think magazines."

"I'm glad someone knows something." She pointed at me, "My companion here doesn't know anything about anything."

With a display of good taste, he ignored her insinuation.

"Bachelorette gifts," she continued. "Movies for sale." She giggled, and I yearned to be anywhere but there.

She looked at the waiter. "Handsome," she said, placing one hand on his arm, "be an angel. Please translate those foreign words for me."

"Kindly wait for me. I'm busy now."

Although the restaurant was good, I never brought her back.

19

A Ghost?

I was lying in bed one night engrossed in the plot of a book, when Mrs. Bromley's loud voice jarred me from my imaginary world.

"Turn the lights off!" she demanded, standing at the threshold of my bedroom. She looked quite angry, and the hatred in her eyes still had the power to upset me.

"Is there something wrong?"

"Turn off the lights."

"I will, but not right now, I'm reading."

"I said, turn the lights off now!" she shouted.

I leapt to my feet. "At least tell me why. What's wrong?"

"Because it's extremely dangerous, that's why."

"What's dangerous?"

"None of your business."

"There's nothing to worry about, Mrs. Bromley." I tried to soothe her fears. "Don't be afraid, I'm with you."

"Hah!" she sneered. "Who's afraid?"

"I mean, nothing's going to happen to you. You're safe."

"Safe? Perhaps. But it's extremely costly for me."

"I don't understand. Will you please explain?"

"You don't pay the electricity, I do." She switched the lights off and strutted out of the room.

For a moment I considered turning them back on, but decided against it, to avoid an argument. I turned on the TV instead. I lowered the volume, but within seconds, she was back, turned off the TV and said, "Are you challenging me? You're absolutely diabolic! Why did you turn on the TV?"

I took a deep breath. "What's wrong with that?"

"You owe me respect. You're here to obey my orders," she said, and walked out of the room.

Apparently I hadn't yet made good on my pledge not to let her offend me—her rudeness still hurt. I reminded myself that I was at her home and she was the one paying the bills, so she had the right. I knew I would have to keep praying for patience in order to deal with her sudden changes of mood. *Virgen de la Caridad, please help.*

Within a few moments she was back.

"Lolita, I want the women in my bedroom to leave. I don't sleep with women. If they were men, it would be different."

"What women?"

"The women who came from upstairs to my bedroom." She motioned for me to follow. "Come and see the boats passing by, with tons of nosy people peeking into my house. I don't want anyone invading my privacy."

"I don't need to see anything, Mrs. Bromley. The women just left. And remember the thick drapes? They give you privacy. Even with all the lights on, people can't see anything inside your house."

"You're smart and I'm stupid? Is that what you're saying?"

I got back in bed and pulled the blankets up to my neck. "Good night, Mrs. Bromley. Sleep tight."

"Of course. If I sleep tight, then you can bring men in your room and keep them all for yourself." She turned on the lights and pointed a finger at me. "If I don't see monkey business in action, how I'm going to remember how it's done? But you are too selfish to let me watch,"

I could hardly believe what she was saying, yet I couldn't stop myself from laughing.

"Yes, ma'am," I said. "Your wish is my command. I'll let you know whenever I find a prospect."

"You have the right to bring men in, because you pay rent—but you don't pay for electricity. It's imperative that the house be completely dark at night. If you don't like that, move out. I have several people lined up for this room. And when you have a man over, make sure you get rent money."

Much later, when I thought she was asleep for the night, I heard the clattering of silverware. I looked at the clock and it was almost two in the morning. I slid on my robe and went to the dining room. Mrs. Bromley was setting up the dining-room table.

"Molly, how nice of you to come. Be an angel and help me. Put the silverware next to the glasses."

"Why? Who's coming?"

"Robert is coming for supper."

"When did he tell you? I haven't seen him around."

"I was sleeping when he pulled my feet and spoke in my ear."

I didn't believe in ghosts, but her words gave me the chills. I knew she was hallucinating, nevertheless, I had an eerie feeling. For an instant, I wanted to go back to bed and cover my head with the blanket, the way I used to do when I was a child. But now I was an adult in charge of a delusional woman who was preparing dinner for a ghost.

Mrs. Bromley was intent on setting the table, so I started putting the knives and forks besides the plates.

"Fold the napkins fancily. Be creative."

I proceeded to fold the napkins in the elegant way I had seen in restaurants.

"You are talented, Molly. They look good. Now, I want to use the silver candlesticks and everything needed for a romantic night. As soon as he gets here, you get out of sight."

"Why? Don't you want me to serve dinner?"

"No. Leave everything ready and then get out of here. But first, chill the champagne."

"But, I want to stay and help."

"I don't need your help; we want to be alone. Maybe this time he will finally have me." She put a vase of flowers on the center of the table and stepped back to appraise her work. "Good. Now I'm going to dress up for him. *Bon nuit*, Molly."

How much I pitied her. I went back to my room, and after a while, I went back to see what she was doing in her bedroom. She had on an evening dress and was sitting in front of the mirror, brushing her hair.

"Why are you still here, Lolita? Disappear!" she said nervously.

This was one of those moments when I wished she were out of it, so I could spare the pain I was about to cause her.

"I'm very sorry, Mrs. Bromley. Robert just called. He said he can't make it tonight, but he'll be here tomorrow morning."

"If you don't have good news, I don't want bad news. Get out."

I left, and in a few moments, she came to my bedroom on the verge of tears.

"What time is he coming tomorrow?"

"Eight in the morning."

By seven the next morning, I wondered why Mrs. Bromley wasn't up. She usually awoke early, with a big smile. It was about the only time of day I enjoyed her because her mean streak hadn't yet surfaced.

I went to her room to check. Since she didn't answer my tapping at the door, I stepped in. Bowdie jumped off the bed to greet me. Mrs. Bromley had the covers pulled up to her face. For a moment I thought she might be dead, and I moved up closer to see if she was breathing.

"Leave me alone," she yelled.

"Are you okay?"

"I want to be alone. Get out!" She sounded like Greta Garbo. Since nothing appeared to be wrong with her, I left.

Two hours later, she was still not up, which worried me. I went to check on her again and smelled something awful as I stood by the door. I thought she or Bowdie had passed gas. When she saw me, she closed her eyes and turned her head away. "Go away and don't come back!"

I moved closer, and the smell became stronger. I thought she hadn't flushed the toilet, so I went in the bathroom to check, but found nothing. I came back to her side and asked, "Mrs. Bromley, would you like your breakfast in bed?"

"Get out of here. Don't you understand English? I want to be alone."

"If you're sick, I need to call the doctor."

"What did you say?"

"I'll call your doctor!" I screamed.

"No!" she yelled, turning toward me.

I assumed she was depressed because Robert didn't show up. "Then I'll take you to the hospital," I said.

"No! I don't want anybody to see me!"

"Why? You look fine."

"I don't care how I look. Go away. I don't want to talk to you, and I'm not going to move from here."

"What's wrong, Mrs. Bromley? Would you like me to call your grandson?" I asked.

She stared at me, and I saw terror in her eyes. "I'm so ashamed. I want to die. Don't tell my grandson. Don't tell anybody what I did."

I felt her anguish; I caressed her cheeks, and I wanted to put my arms around her and brush away her fears. "No, I won't tell anyone, but you have to trust me. Please tell me what's upsetting you. I want to help."

"Lolita, how could this happen to me? I'm…"

I waited for her to go on, but she didn't volunteer any further information.

"You are what? Please tell me what happened, so I can help you."

She closed her lips tightly and said nothing.

"Would you please tell me what you are afraid of, for God's sake?"

She turned her head aside.

"Mrs. Bromley please, I'll understand, no matter what's troubling you."

"Nothing! Get out!"

"I'll leave, but I'll be back with your grandson."

She looked at me with teary eyes. She looked so vulnerable that my heart cried for her.

"*Mon Dieu*," she cried, tossing the blanket off of her. "There. Are you satisfied? I'm swimming in my own *merde*!"

I was nauseated. She was covered in diarrhea, and it was all over the bed. I covered my mouth and raced to the bathroom, barely in time to lose my breakfast. I quickly splashed water on my face and struggled to gain my composure. I wondered how I was going to handle this situation. I had endurance for a lot of things in life, but diarrhea wasn't one of them. It had been difficult for me to change diapers when my children were small, and most of the time it had turned my stomach. I didn't want to embarrass Mrs. Bromley any more than she already was by vomiting while cleaning her up, so I thought of calling a nurse's aide to help. I knew this was not possible, but I had to do something before it hardened on her. It was urgent that I do something, yet I stood frozen. Finally, I recalled Mrs. Bromley saying many times in the past, "*Let's get it over with*." Having no other choice, I tied a bandanna doused with cologne across my face, put on disposable gloves, and prayed for God's help, so I wouldn't get sick. I made the signal of the cross and held my breath.

I approached Mrs. Bromley with a large washbasin. She looked at me wide-eyed, obviously frightened.

"Lolita, why do you have that across your face? Am I having surgery?"

"No, dear. I'm going to clean you up, that's all. Relax."

"I beg of you, please, don't tell Robert about this, or he'll never try to make love to me. Will you promise?"

I realized that my struggles with Mrs. Bromley were strengthening my will, but unfortunately Alzheimer's was breaking hers.

20

Suffocated

The new Spanish semester began, and Jane followed through with her promise to take care of Mrs. Bromley on Wednesdays, so I could continue teaching my class. Each time I returned, Jane let off steam by telling me how much she disliked Mrs. Bromley.

"Betty was always so haughty," Jane would say. "She made my life miserable when I was married to her son, and now I still have to put up with all of this."

I was glad that Jane confided in me. It helped me understand why she was so antagonistic toward her mother-in-law.

One Wednesday when I arrived, she was nervously pacing the living room. I left my bag on the floor and sat on the couch.

"You don't look well today, Jane," I said hesitantly.

"Believe it or not, Betty was so naughty in the restaurant today that I cut short our lunch and left the restaurant."

"I'm sorry, Jane."

"I'm sorry too, but there's nothing we can do. I gave her a sedative and tucked her in bed, otherwise I would have suffered a breakdown." She sat next to me. "You know, Lolita, I get here filled with the best of intentions. I try to forget the past and be kind to her, but she always manages to bring out the worst in me. All my good intentions turn to anger and frustration." She pushed her hair back from her face and continued, "At the end of the day, she still has the power to make my life miserable. I despise her as much now as I did then, and I have no respect for her. What's worse, I don't respect myself either for having these hateful feelings. I don't care if she is sick, and I don't know how you can deal with her every day and night, seven days a week."

"It's my job, Jane. I force myself to remember that she doesn't want to be mean. She can't help the way she is because of her terrible disease. Try to be patient."

"I ran out of patience. She's crazy! She has always been!" Jane yelled. "She's evil. She manipulate us. She belittles us. I can't believe you defend her."

I was dumbfounded. It frightened me to think what Jane might do, carrying so much hate.

"Jane," I said, "I don't understand your reaction. You know she is sick. You are with her only one day of the week, can't you just ignore her and pay no attention to what she says?"

"Easy for you to say, your heart isn't full of resentment," Jane confessed. "She had always been impossible to get along with and had always made my life miserable, because she thought I wasn't good enough for her son."

I really wanted to discuss the matter further but decided against it. I thought it would be better to mind my own business, but I found it hard to do, because I had grown fond of Mrs. Bromley. Even if it was a love-hate relationship, there was a very special place in my heart for her.

I was surprised of Jane's temper; something told me not to ever cross her path.

The following Wednesday, Jane handed me a piece of paper. "Since you like to write," she said, "I wrote a profile of Betty. Just a few lines will tell you what she is."

I read the words aloud. "Mrs. Elizabeth Bromley is a woman who has banked on her good looks and small talk all her life. She never acquired any interests and never acquired an intelligent approach to fill the void in her life, which grew larger and larger even before she had her first face-lift. Lolita, if you ever write about her, you need to show her character: mean, haughty, and arrogant, with a streak of selfishness in every thing she does."

I thought the characterization was exaggerated. Not having known Mrs. Bromley before her illness, the list of unflattering attributes left me sad because I knew there was some truth to it.

I thought that if I were to write a book about Mrs. Bromley, the book would be about the effects of Alzheimer's on caregivers and families and the importance of understanding the bizarre behavior displayed by its victims.

As I continued to observe the disease closely, I relished the fleeting moments of awareness, as they became sparser. I basked on those short moments of lucidity to let her know she was loved and cared for. She might never appreciate it, but I felt at peace with myself.

I remembered one night when Mrs. Bromley was awake and dressed up at ten at night, ready to go to mass with me. I tried to convince her that church was closed, but to no avail. Her mind was set on going, no matter what. I had no other choice but to drive her to church. I went as far as trying to open the doors. All of them were locked. As we drove back home, she kept repeating: "God knows it isn't my fault we couldn't get in. I don't want to be punished. I do not want to go to hell."

Another time she insisted that I take her to the bank, even though it was Sunday. She said she had an appointment with the manager. Again I took her and tried the locked doors. She blamed me for making her late. The same thing happened when she insisted she had an appointment with the hairdresser. We went there and were informed that she didn't have an appointment that day. Characteristically, after each of those episodes, she became subdued for a while.

My daughter Leti's new job made it impossible for her to cover for me, even on Saturdays, which made it impossible for me to attend my writers' group. I missed the interaction with other writers.

I asked Mr. Williams for Saturdays off. He began to search for a part-time companion, but none of those he interviewed were right for the job. I knew it would be difficult, so I decided to find someone myself. I thought of Meri, my Mexican dancer friend who had recently retired. Of course, it would work. They had dancing and show-business in common, so they could enjoy each other's company while reminiscing about their performing days.

I was right. Meri eagerly accepted, and Mr. Williams was delighted. Upon my advice, Meri brought along clippings, photos, and some outfits from her dancing shows, which caused Mrs. Bromley to be taken with her at once. Her past sprang from within, and she opened the black trunk where she tenderly housed her fondest memories of bygone days. It helped her to reminisce on a time she loved. Everything seemed to be working fine.

For several weeks, I returned on Saturday evenings to find an energetic Mrs. Bromley, her eyes sparkling with new emotion. One time I found her wearing an evening gown with a long train and a wide-brimmed hat.

High spirited, she said, "I'm going to the Easter Parade."

I applauded, and she bowed, displaying a charming, genuine smile.

The peaceful and happy times went on for a while, until gradually it began to fade and the two women started to get on each other's nerves.

One evening when I opened the front door, I found Meri kneeling down in the hallway, massaging the dog's neck. "What happened to Bowdie?" I asked.

"Mrs. Bromley almost killed the poor thing," Meri answered in a faltering voice. "I think she's okay now; at least she can keep her head up. I've been talking to her and massaging her neck."

"How? What on earth did she do?"

"Mrs. Bromley was walking the dog in the front yard when a big dog ran by; Bowdie broke loose and rushed into the street. With surprising agility, the old bat went after her and brought the dog back to the yard."

"Did the other dog attack Bowdie?"

"No. But Mrs. Bromley was mad, and she got Bowdie by its neck and dangled her in the air until she began to suffocate. The evil woman flung the poor thing to the ground and Bowdie went limp. 'Mrs. Bromley,' I cried out, 'you almost killed your dog!' 'Well, she has to die of something!' she snapped back. 'But you said you loved her,' I said. She replied, 'I will not tolerate disobedience and that's final. You ought to remember that yourself!'"

"Oh, Meri," I said as I caressed Bowdie. "That was awful! The poor thing."

With tears in her eyes, Meri said, "Look, thank God the dog is coming to."

"Lolitaaa!" Mrs. Bromley shouted from the living room.

"That's for me," Meri said. "She calls me Lolita."

"Don't worry, she'll call you Meri soon. She still calls me Molly most of the time."

"*Ay, chihuahua*, I don't care. But I hope I won't be here long enough for her to call me by my name."

"Lolitaaa…!"

"Stay with Bowdie. I'll go," I said and called out, "Coming, Mrs. Bromley."

"It's about time. I've been calling."

"Meri and I are taking care of Bowdie," I interrupted.

"Did she die?" she asked calmly.

"How can you be so callous?" I looked at her. "It's your so called baby who could be dying, you know."

"She's old. We all have to die someday. Maybe her time has come."

"How can you talk like that? You said Bowdie meant everything to you."

"Of course she does." Suddenly, the color drained from her face. She hurried to the hallway. Meri was stroking the dog. "My treasure," she cooed. "What's wrong with you? Baby, come to mama."

"Oh, no. Don't you touch her!" Meri cried out.

"It's okay, Meri," I said.

Mrs. Bromley bent down and lifted the dog.

"Don't let her, Lolita. She'll kill the poor thing."

"Meri, she's okay now. Don't provoke her."

Mrs. Bromley grabbed my arm. "*Mon Dieu*, let's take baby to the hospital at once."

I touched her shoulder. "Bowdie will be just fine. Let her rest for awhile. It's all she needs for now."

"Let's give her some water," Meri said. "I think she's thirsty."

"Whatever you say, darling." She turned to Meri. "You did a good job with my treasure. We have to give the devil his due. For once this woman has done something right."

Bowdie recuperated, but we engaged in a new battle. Even though the veterinarian put Bowdie on a very strict diet, Mrs. Bromley insisted on feeding her fattening fried foods and desserts from her own plate. Trying to break this habit, I started a routine of serving Mrs. Bromley dinner first; while she ate, I'd take the dog for a walk. Before leaving, I'd explain to her, "Mrs. Bromley, while you eat, I'm taking Bowdie for a walk."

"Good idea," she'd answer, but soon she would be looking for us.

I tried locking Bowdie in one of the bathrooms while she ate, but she would let her out. Tying the dog on the back porch didn't work either. She would always stop eating to look for Bowdie.

One morning she came to my bedroom with Bowdie wrapped in a towel.

"She is throwing up! She's dying! Don't stand there doing nothing! Hurry! Let us go to the hospital."

I jumped up, got dressed, and grabbed the car keys. "She'll be all right. Don't worry."

"My poor baby, hang in there! Even if you are old, don't die. Please, don't die! Do not leave me alone!"

In order to run some tests, the veterinarian asked to keep Bowdie overnight. On the way home we stopped for breakfast, and Mrs. Bromley told everyone in the restaurant about Bowdie being hospitalized.

I started to read a newspaper, which she obviously didn't like. "You are oblivious to the pain of my darling Bowdie," she said, drumming her fingers on the table. "Besides, it is not polite to read in front of me."

"I'm only scanning the paper, and I am very concerned for Bowdie. Don't you know that you are to blame?"

"You just put your foot in your mouth again. If you cannot say something nice, do not say anything at all."

"But I know what I'm saying. You feed Bowdie all the wrong foods. I know you don't mean it, but you're killing her."

"I am what?"

"You keep ignoring the fact that the doctor put her on a special diet. She's very old. Her liver is enlarged, her heart isn't working right, not to mention she's too fat… Every night we fight because of the unhealthy food you feed her. All the sweets you give her are killing her."

"I didn't know that." She scratched her chin and avoided my eyes. "Why doesn't anybody ever tell me anything? I'm the last one to find out what's going on."

"Will you remember from now on not to feed he from your plate and to only feed her the special food?"

"What special food?"

"I'll show it to you again when we get home. Meanwhile, I want you to write down, with your own handwriting, that you are not to feed Bowdie anything but her own food, and keep it in your purse."

For a moment she appeared flustered. "Just in case I forget, would you write a note for my purse?"

"That's what I just told you, but you write it yourself so you will recognize your handwriting. That way you will know that you agreed."

"Well, you should have said so. Before you spoke gibberish. How could I understand?"

"Okay, dear Mrs. Bromley. Whatever you say."

"When are we picking up Bowdie?"

"We just left her at the vet's. She's spending the night there."

"The night? Why?"

"They need to run tests and do blood work."

"There's absolutely nothing wrong with her. The only thing they want to do is bleed me. My money, that's what everybody wants."

Poor rich woman, money's all you think about. Although you have it, you can't buy an ounce of sanity.

The next morning, Mrs. Bromley showed up at my doorstep, all dressed up. "Lolita, wake up, we're going to pick up my darling Bowdie."

I rubbed my eyes and looked at the time. "It's too early, the place is closed."

"Move, sleepyhead. Call to see how she spent the night. Go on! Tell them we are on our way to pick her up."

I made the call, knowing she wouldn't leave my room otherwise.

She came closer and pointed a finger at me. "How come you hung up the phone without talking?"

"It was a recording. Somebody will be there at eight."

"Nobody cares about Bowdie. Who knows what those sadists have put her through? I want to see her now."

"Will you please be kind enough to wait for me in the living room while I get ready?"

"*Bon*. Hurry! Do not take a shower, and remember that I'm waiting. Tra la la la. Tra la la," she sang her way to the living room.

When driving by Saint John's Church, I suggested a visit to God's house.

"Good idea," she said. "We need to pray for Bowdie's health."

After church, hoping she had forgotten about going to see Bowdie, I drove back home.

"What are we doing back here?" she demanded as I parked in front of her house.

"We're home."

"Smartass! I know we are home. What are we doing here? That's what I want to know!"

"I'm going to prepare a nice meal. It's past our breakfast time you know." I tried to sound convincing, but her eyes narrowed and she glared at me.

"Take me to pick up Bowdie. Immediately!"

"Yes, ma'am, at once," I said, knowing I couldn't trick her this time.

I drove to the veterinary clinic and she was out of the car before I could put it in park. Again Mrs. Bromley surprised me with her agility. It was like she had left behind the pain and aches of old age.

She pushed the door open and walked up to the receptionist. "I demand to see Bowdie right this moment!"

The receptionist looked at her and said in a conciliatory tone, "Good morning, Mrs. Bromley. Please, have a seat."

"Don't good-morning me, and don't play smart. I want to see Bowdie right now!" she roared.

Attracted by the commotion, the veterinarian appeared and approached her. "Mrs. Bromley, it's nice to see you." He took her hand. "Come on. We'll go see Bowdie. She's resting now."

I was confident that in the presence of a man, she'd be more than content. When she returned, she looked radiant.

"Lolita, we can go now. Bowdie is in the hands of a very charming doctor. He explained that Bowdie needs to stay longer and I acquiesced. And do you know what? He found me very attractive."

21

Police

It was another classic Florida hot sunny day in July. I felt especially good because the students from my Spanish class had expressed their appreciation by holding a little pre-birthday party for me in the classroom. The handmade cards they gave me were filled with heartfelt messages. I was very proud of the group, and a sense of satisfaction filled my heart with the realization that the goals I had set when I began the course had been achieved.

When I got home later that day, I found a message to call Jane immediately. I made the call, my high spirits quickly deflated.

Jane's tone of immediacy scared me. "Lolita," she said, "you need to get over here right away, so I can leave. Or else I'm going to commit murder."

"What happened?" I asked, dreading what I might hear.

"I'm at the end of my rope. I'm completely out of patience, and I don't want to do something I'll regret later."

"Calm down. What's going on?"

"You won't believe it." Jane cleared her throat. "I was on the phone when Betty told me to stop blabbering. I told her to be patient and wait until I finished. She mimicked me. Then, she stuck her tongue out. I asked her to stop her nonsense. Then she actually spit in my face."

"Oh, how awful—"

"I couldn't help it and slapped her face. She grabbed my hand. We struggled, and I shoved her against the wall. I hate myself for letting her bring out the worst in me."

"Please, Jane, calm down."

"I despise that woman! I need to get out of here, get her out of my sight. I can't cope with the guilt I feel for hating her so much."

"But Jane," I said, trying to console her, "don't torture yourself. She'll forget the whole thing very soon."

"You are not getting my point!" Jane snapped. "She'll forget, but I won't!"

140

"I'm sorry. I really don't know what else to say."

Jane coughed nervously. "I know, Lolita. I'm sorry. This situation is very touchy. Please come over right now?"

"I'm on my way."

By the time I got there, Jane had left. Mrs. Bromley seemed glad to see me and didn't waste any time showing me the bruises on her arms, which I hoped would fade away soon, since they looked suspicious and people might think I abused her.

The next morning during breakfast I reminded her, "Mrs. Bromley, you know that we need to be out of the house by ten?"

She looked surprised. "How am I suppose to know if no one tells me anything? Why do we have to leave?"

"Because the exterminator is coming to spray the house for bugs, and we have to be out."

"That's new. Why doesn't anyone tell me what's going on in my own house? Certainly, my baby is coming too."

"Oh, yes. We won't leave Bowdie, she has to be out too."

"For how long exactly."

"Four hours."

"What am I going to do for four hours?"

"You're going to the beauty parlor to make yourself beautiful."

"What do you mean?" she asked.

I touched her hair lightly. "Linda will do your hair, Wanda will do your nails, and Irene will give you a pedicure."

"But it will take too long. Where's Bowdie going to be?" she inquired, as if this were the first time she had been through this routine.

"She will be in her beauty salon too. The girl that grooms your baby adores her. She knows how to make the little rascal look embraceable."

"You mean clean, because she's always embraceable and beautiful."

"Well, her fur will shine still more."

She smiled. "Lolita, you are not dumb. In fact, you are very clever."

I smiled back. "Why?"

"Because I like the way you run my house."

The exterminator arrived promptly at ten. Mrs. Bromley met him at the door, smiling, and Bowdie barked incessantly. I ran behind, trying to stop the barking.

"Baby, it is all right," Mrs. Bromley said. "This good man will get rid of your fleas. Would you come in, please?"

"Thank you, lady. I'll begin outside."

"Whatever you wish," she said, following him into the front yard.

I hurried inside the house to pick up the bag with the things we needed. I was back in five minutes and saw Mrs. Bromley whispering something to the exterminator. I didn't think anything of it and helped her and Bowdie into the car.

At eight the next morning, there was a loud thumping at the door. I looked through the window and saw the gate open and a police car parked outside the gate. I ran to the door and opened it.

"Good morning, officer," I said. "May I help you?"

"Are you Mrs. Bromley?"

"No, I'm her companion." Although I was puzzled, I tried not to show any concern. "Why do you want to see her so early?" I asked.

"It's police business. Is Mrs. Elizabeth Bromley here?"

"Yes, but she's not up yet." I knew that I had to notify Mr. Williams first. "Will you please come back around noon, if you want to talk to her?"

He glanced at his watch. "We'll be back at ten. Have her ready to talk to us by then."

As soon as they left, I called Mr. Williams and explained what had happened. In ten minutes he was at the door.

"Do you know what the police wanted?" he asked right away.

"I have no idea, but I'm afraid she's going to be scared to see the police in her house," I said.

"I'll talk to her first. Is she in her room?"

A few minutes later, he returned with Mrs. Bromley, still in her robe.

"Grandmere, please sit here," he said, helping her onto the couch. "Let's have a cup of coffee and chat a little bit."

"*Mon Dieu*! This is something new…but I'm not complaining."

I brought them each a cup of coffee.

"The police want to talk to you," Mr. Williams said.

"About what?" she asked.

"Oh probably about buying tickets for a raffle, so no need to be nervous."

She grinned." Why would I be nervous? I haven't killed anybody yet. How about you? If you did, we can blame it on Lolita."

Mr. Williams and I laughed.

At ten sharp, the two officers returned. I showed them into the living room. On seeing them, Mrs. Bromley started to rise.

"I'm Officer Ken Barnet and this is Officer Mark Brown," one of the police-men said, signaling for her not to stand. "Please don't get up."

"That will be the day, when I stay still in the presence of two handsome young men."

Unmoved, he replied, "We just want you to be comfortable."

"I am fine, thank you." She flashed the kind of smile she used when flirting. "Now, officers, what can I do for you? How about a drink?" She turned to me. "Lolita, see what they want to drink. Maybe scotch, brandy, or—"

Officer Brown interrupted. "No, thank you Mrs. Bromley, we're on duty. We need to ask you a few questions."

"I'm sorry, handsome. I didn't mean to offend you." She folded her hands on her lap and continued, "Ask me anything and I will do my best to comply."

"We're here to help you." Officer Barnet said, leaning toward her. "Has some-one been mistreating you?"

"What are you talking about?" she shouted.

Officer Barnet held up his hand. "Don't be upset, Mrs. Bromley. Perhaps you don't want to talk in front of so many people?"

Mr. Williams, the color drained from his face, leaped to his feet. "Wait one minute, what's going on? I'm her grandson, and this is Lolita Rimblas, her abso-lutely trustworthy full-time companion."

"Do you have any objections if we speak with your grandmother alone?"

Mr. Williams frowned and thought for a moment. "Go ahead! But I'd like to know what the problem is."

"We're looking into an elderly-abuse complaint," Officer Brown explained.

"Complaint? From whom? I make sure my grandmother has the best care in the world."

"That very well may be…but it's my duty to investigate any complaints."

Mr. Williams couldn't hide his annoyance. "I suppose I have the right to know who filed such a complaint."

"Sorry. I'm not allowed to reveal that…but Mrs. Bromley said she's been con-stantly abused by a woman."

Mr. Williams was about to explode, but he held back his rage. "That's a lie!"

"We want a doctor to examine her," the officer replied.

Oh heavens, I thought, *what if they blame me for her bruises?* I would be the most obvious suspect.

"I commend you for taking the elderly-abuse issue so seriously," Mr. Williams told the officers, "but I think you should investigate the case before alarming peo-ple. Look, my grandmother is ninety-years-old and suffers from Alzheimer's. She has delusions and short-term memory loss. Check with her doctor. I don't think you can get anything reliable from her."

"I understand all that, but we still need to ask her some questions," said officer Brown. "So if you and Miss Rimblas will step out of the room, we can get this over with."

Mr. Williams sighed, "If that's what you want."

Mr. Williams and I started to leave, but Mrs. Bromley called me back. "Molly, I want you to stay."

"Is it okay for me to stay?" I asked. The officer nodded. I walked back into the room and sat on the sofa.

"Mrs. Bromley," the younger man asked, "may we see your arms?"

"You certainly can." She began to raise her sleeve.

"Do you wish Miss Rimblas to help you?"

She shook her head. "Officer, who's Miss Rimblas? I don't need help. I'm not that old. I may be pushing sixty, but I'm perfectly capable of doing my own things."

I suppressed a laugh, remembering the many times she had lied about her age.

The officer examined her arms. "Do you have any other bruises?"

"You may look for yourself." She started unbuttoning her robe, but the officer stopped her.

"We'll send a female officer to examine you. But first tell us how you got these bruises. Did anyone hurt you?"

She laughed. "I thought you were here to investigate. You tell me who did it."

The two officers looked at each other.

"Of course we are," Officer Brown said. "We want you to be safe while we find out how you got those bruises."

She clasped her hands to her head. "Please do. I don't remember, but I want you to find out who is beating me."

"Don't you worry," he said. "We assure you that we'll look into it."

"How do I know I can trust you?"

"You can trust us. We're going to talk to your grandson and we'll clear this up," said Officer Burnet.

They both shook her hand and headed for the door. I followed them.

"Will you please call Mr. Williams?" Officer Brown said.

I fetched Mr. Williams, and they all walked out of the house.

When Mr. Williams returned, Mrs. Bromley had gone to her room.

"Lolita," he said, "the exterminator was the one who complained because my grandmother asked him to."

"Yes, Mr. Williams, I thought so. It happened in the five minutes that I left her alone to get my things, when I returned she was whispering to the exterminator."

"With her, that's all the time she needs to get in trouble."

I recalled the day she had been waiting in the restaurant to talk to Bryan. That time it took only one minute.

"I convinced those two that nothing was wrong here. I explained how easily she bruises, and that just by holding her arms to help her in or out of a chair might do it."

22

Coquettish

For days, Mrs. Bromley closely followed the development of her bruises as they darkened and grew in size. She wanted to know how it had happened. I insisted that I didn't know.

Jane didn't show up for several weeks, so I couldn't teach my Spanish class.

Finally, one day Jane called. "Lolita, I got over Betty's episode and I feel guilty about you missing your classes. If you need me, I'm ready to come back."

"Thank you, Jane. I really appreciate it."

I called the center and was able to resume my teaching.

Days passed by and little by little I became melancholic. I began to miss my own home, my own things, and the mementos that make a house a home. I longed for the warmth of my family.

One Saturday I invited Mrs. Bromley to go for a ride to visit my family, even though I knew that Leti and Japhlet were away for the weekend. As always, she was happy to go, as long as Bowdie came along. We embarked on the mini-adventure of driving to my home.

As we got out of the car, my next-door neighbors came over to greet me. Marilyn gave me a hug. "It is so good to see you, Lolita. We miss you."

"Me too. I've been very busy. May I introduce you to Mrs. Bromley? Mrs. Bromley, these nice people are my neighbors, Marilyn and Dave. Would you all like to come in for a cold drink?"

"Lolita," Mrs. Bromley interrupted, "don't you think you should ask me first?"

"Why would I ask you first?" I said. "This is my home."

"Because we are on my time," she answered.

"And what exactly do you mean by your time?" I asked, knowing that something was brewing. The explanation came with her usual despotic reasoning.

"I'm paying you, so therefore your time is mine."

"Why don't you try to be more specific? I still don't understand."

"You should ask first if it's suitable for me to share my time with your friends," she said loudly. "Is it clear enough now? Do you understand?"

I knew I shouldn't argue with her, but her bravado infuriated me and I felt the need to put her in her place. "Now listen to me, Mrs. Bromley—"

"Lolita," Dave interrupted, "don't trouble yourself on our account. We need to get going anyway."

"Please, Dave, don't leave, I beg you to come in," I said. Then I turned to Mrs. Bromley and said, "Mrs. Bromley, today is Sunday. I'm supposed to have the day off. Since there is no one else who will put up with you, I agreed to work so you wouldn't be alone and miserable. But believe me, I'd rather be with my kind and thoughtful friends—"

"So I should thank you," she interrupted.

"Of course not. Just be considerate and let us visit in peace. You can watch TV while we talk. We have a lot of catching up to do."

She bowed graciously. "Please, your majesty, be kind enough to take care of Bowdie first, then be free to entertain your friends."

I picked up Bowdie and we all went inside. We sat in the living room, which overlooked the ocean. I opened the sliding doors so Bowdie could go outside.

"Marilyn, do you mind giving me a hand in the kitchen?"

"Gladly."

I turned to Dave and winked. "I leave you in good company. We'll be right back."

Once in the kitchen, Marilyn commented, "Mrs. Bromley is a character. I have never seen her up close, but she's intimidating, to say the least."

"Did I tell you that she suffers from Alzheimer's?"

"I thought you told me dementia."

"She suffers from both, I think. It's horrible."

"Is Dave safe with her?"

"She loves men. She's on her best behavior when a man is around. That's why I left her with him. I think in her younger years she used to chase men."

We arranged some cheese, crackers, and glasses on a tray, at the same time catching up on the latest events in our lives.

When we returned to the living room, Dave was laughing and Mrs. Bromley was glowing.

"…All of them came to the nightclub to see me dance," she was saying. "Oh, la, la, the memories…" She looked at Marilyn. "This isn't the way to take care of a husband. He's been flirting with me, and I'm about to take him up on his offer to take me out."

We couldn't help but laugh.

"Laugh all you want," Mrs. Bromley went on, "but he can't hide the fact that he's taken by me. There's no way to deny it, and that's all I have to say."

"What's important here is: do you like him?" Marilyn said.

"I'm so used to men's flattery that it doesn't make any difference if I like him or not." She turned to me and added, "Lolita, write down his phone number, just in case I need a man. One never knows."

We had a lively afternoon and laughed endlessly as we listened to Mrs. Bromley's interesting stories. It was the first time my friends were exposed to her, and they enjoyed her spontaneity; at the same time, Mrs. Bromley was in heaven being the center of our attention.

We ate, drank, and laughed a lot. Slowly we got involved in our own interests and started to neglect Mrs. Bromley. She picked up Bowdie and started her own conversation with the dog.

"You're the only faithful friend," she said. "Look at them, talking nonsense and ignoring me. They know nothing about good manners. They're as rude as they come. And look at Lolita. She's the worst…"

Watching through the sliding doors we were absorbed by the magnificent sunset. Soon we leaped to our feet, as if pulled up by springs, to better watch the last strokes of nature's masterpiece.

"Mrs. Bromley, come with us to watch the sunset," I said…

"I don't waste my time in futilities."

"Okay, it's your loss," I said, and turned to enjoy the view.

When we got back to Mrs. Bromley, her change of mood was evident. She sat erect, her face somber.

It was getting dark, so I switched on the lights.

"Turn off the lights!" Mrs. Bromley yelled. "The party is over!"

I was stupefied. "This is not possible," I said, exasperated by her nerve.

"Of course it is possible!" she yelled again.

"Mrs. Bromley, with you, anything is possible," I responded. "What I can't believe is that this is happening to me, again, and in my own house."

On the way back home, I was too upset to talk.

Mrs. Bromley chatted with Bowdie. "What a hellish terrible day Lolita put us through. Imagine, she is a mere ordinary employee!"

After some more babbling, she began to snore. Mrs. Bromley's words: *lights out* had triggered the memory of a nightmare my ex-husband put me through twenty-five years earlier.

Mauricio was a typical macho man, and I was a submissive wife who was terrified of his temper. Even though I had everything money could buy, I lived as a prisoner in my own home. But three times a year, on my children's birthdays, I had the freedom to do anything I wanted to make their parties unforgettable. On those days only, the house was open for all their school mates, siblings and parents. Usually, the fiestas began at noon and lasted until very late at night. I hired clowns and catered all kinds of food. Often the swimming pool would be covered with flowers delivered from Xochimilco, a well-known wholesale place two hours away. Even the media covered the events.

One particular year, it was my youngest daughter Leti's birthday, and I wanted the singer Tito Guizar to entertain. His TV program was the highlight of the week for me; it fueled a crush I'd had on him since I was ten years old.

Leti told her father that she wanted Tito Guizar and his mariachis to sing "Las Mañanitas," the Mexican birthday song, for her at the party.

"He is too old to sing for children," Mauricio said. "Call someone else proper for your age."

Leti insisted until her father gave in.

Mauricio had been jealous of Tito forever, so he suspected that I was behind Leti's wishes.

I found out the name of Tito's tailor and had Leti fitted for a *charro* outfit exactly like the one Tito was to use at the party. The invitations were designed with pictures of Leti and Tito in identical outfits.

On the day of the party, my husband never came out to meet the singer. Before Tito began the first show, he asked for Mauricio and was told that *Señor* Rimblas was playing poker with his friends in the studio. Tito asked to join them in between breaks, but my husband answered: "Tell that singer he doesn't have enough money to play at my table."

When the time arrived for the last performance, it seemed Tito wanted to get even with my husband's rudeness and used my name, Lolita, in songs with female names. The songs were heard all over the house. I was so embarrassed that I wanted the ground to open up and swallow me. When the show was over, the guests seemed delighted as they praised Tito for his performance.

Since Tito didn't want supper until he had finished performing, I asked the maid to have the dining room ready for the performers when the last show was over.

I escorted the guests that hadn't had dinner to the dining room. Soon after we sat down to eat, the lights went off. We thought it was a momentary electrical shortage. The remaining older children, still enjoying themselves in the garden, came running into the house.

Eduardo, our chauffeur, entered the dining room and declared, "On behalf of Don Mauricio I must turn the lights off because the party is over!"

Suddenly, Mrs. Bromley's voice brought me back. "Lolita, why did you let me sleep in the car like one of those old people having catnaps everywhere?" she asked sleepily.

Several days later, Leti and Japhlet showed up. Surprised, I greeted them at the front door.

"*Hola*, Japhlet, Leti. Thank you for coming," I said as I opened the door. "Come right in."

"Although you insisted on not going," said Leti hugging me, "I know how important Joe's wedding is for you. And please, *Mamita*, don't tell me that you are not going, because that's why we are here."

"I told you I don't want—" I began, and Leti interrupted.

"Not a word. Go...get ready. Take your time and make yourself beautiful."

"Okay. I know Mrs. Bromley is happy when you and Japhlet stay with her, so I have nothing to worry about. Now go to her while I get dressed."

Once I was ready, I went to the living room to say good-bye.

Mrs. Bromley clapped her hands. "*Mon Dieu*!" she exclaimed. "Look at Lolita! She looks like a movie star. I'm sure you're going to look better than the bride, so don't you dare come back here without the best catch in the party. Gorgeous!"

I was at a loss for words, but I managed to say, "Thank you, Mrs. Bromley. Coming from you, I believe every word you say."

"To complete your look, wear my mink coat."

"I appreciate it, but it's too hot."

"Then use my jewelry."

"Thank you kindly, but it's too dangerous. I don't want to be mugged on account of your jewelry."

I couldn't believe the change in Mrs. Bromley, she was actually offering me her valuables. I never expected to live long enough to see such a metamorphosis. Not since our visit to Leti's school has she shown that much kindness towards me.

23

Violence

"Hi ho, hi ho, it's off to work I go. La, la, la, la…" I sang the tune from *Snow White and the Seven Dwarfs* as I drove to work at the end of my day off. Lately, I had been looking forward to seeing Mrs. Bromley, who for a change had been easy to control.

Meri and Mrs. Bromley kept busy talking about past performances and exchanging newspaper clippings from their golden days. They dressed up in costumes to do their dancing numbers. Meri preferred to stay home rather than going out like Leti and Japhlet used to do.

I stood at the front door and turned the key. As I walked in, I was horrified to see my CD stand and broken CDs all over the floor. I froze. Strewn in front of me was my collection of classical music that had lifted my spirits during hours of writing. As I picked one up, my anger soared. It was *Sweet Mystery of Life*, by Jeanette MacDonald and Nelson Eddy.

"What happened?" I asked.

Meri rushed toward me and pointed at the floor. "I didn't clean up, so you could see the mess."

"Who did this?"

"You need to ask? Who else?"

"But for heaven's sake, why?"

"Mrs. Bromley was in a rage and knocked over your CD stand, then she threw the CDs at me and the wall. I tried to stop her, but she pushed me away. That old bat has the strength of a bull. I asked her to pick up the CDs, but she refused. You should have seen the wrath in her eyes. I demanded an apology, but she refused to do that too."

Anger blinded me, and I wanted to hit something. I was mad at Meri for allowing it to happen. It was absurd to ask a crazy woman to apologize. With a deep sigh, I managed to ask, "What triggered it?"

"Well, after her nap, she dressed up and wanted to go to a nice place for afternoon tea."

"Why didn't you take her? That's part of her routine."

"She spent all her money at lunch and I didn't have any with me. I tried to explain that neither of us had money. She produced some English pounds from her purse and waved them in my face."

"When did she begin throwing my CDs at you? That's what I want to know, because she doesn't have fits unless she's provoked."

"She insisted on going, so I stood in front of the door and refused to let her out. That's when she flung a CD case at me, followed by some more. I reached for her hand, but she pushed me and I almost fell. She kept throwing the stupid cases at me with all her might. Then she told me to pick them up. I told her that since she was the one who made the mess, she should pick them up. She stomped on each CD and said that I was pay to clean up after her. I told her that if she didn't apologize, I'd quit and leave her alone. She laughed and pointed to the door. Oh, Lolita, I don't want to see her ever again!"

Faced with the possibility of losing Meri, my anger was replaced by fear.

"You're not quitting, are you?" I asked. She didn't answer. Finally, Meri spoke. "I've lost all respect for Mrs. Bromley. I'm really furious."

"We know her dementia takes over most of the time," I said. "That's why we shouldn't argue. It's safer and easier to play along with her outbursts."

"You're too lenient. She's more spoiled than sick."

"Nevertheless, Meri, she doesn't have it all together. I shouldn't have left my CDs out. She's like a child, so our duty is to avoid a crisis before it happens."

"How can I avoid a crisis if I can't tell when one is coming? Her conversation is smart and makes a lot of sense; then, without warning, a tantrum begins."

"That was my problem too, but now I know she's not herself when she gets angry. She's really sick," I said.

"I'm sorry, but I don't care. I don't want to take care of her again. I'll help you clean up this mess before I leave."

We proceeded to clean up, trying to salvage as many CDs as possible. To my surprise, Meri did this in silence. This was unusual for her because her words always came at you nonstop, like a machine gun.

After Meri left, I wanted to check on Mrs. Bromley, but I needed time to cool off. It concerned me that her door was closed and I didn't see any lights under the door. When my anger subsided, I knocked on the door.

"Mrs. Bromley, may I come in?"

When she didn't respond to several of my attempts, I opened the door and turned on the light. The scene in front of me broke my heart. Mrs. Bromley was kneeling on the floor, hunched over the side of the bed. I approached her and placed my hand on her shoulder.

"Mrs. Bromley, are you okay?" I asked.

She gasped and looked up. Her eyes seemed unfocused as she searched my face. I knelt down beside her and reached for her hand. "Are you okay?"

She looked at me, her gaze an eternity of confusion. All I felt was pity.

I hurried to the kitchen for a warm glass of milk and coaxed her to drink it. Then I helped her into her nightgown and tucked her into bed. I was deeply affected by what I had seen. I preferred the boisterous and outspoken Mrs. Bromley to the wretched woman in front of me.

Back in my bedroom, the defeated attitude of Mrs. Bromley as well as the gloominess surrounding the room, reminded me of a similar scene a long time ago.

It was a cheerful, bright day during lunch. I was discussing a matter with my husband, who didn't like to be contradicted. To avoid violent scenes in front of the children, I always gave in, but this particular day, I wanted the children to know that I had a mind of my own. I stood my ground and defended my point of view, showing courage I didn't know I had. Suddenly, he grabbed a watermelon from the table and threw it with all his might against the wall. The fruit exploded and splattered all over, onto the ceiling and drapes. For weeks, I could still see seeds of the fruit in the dining room as a reminder of his violence, probably like I would find traces of the broken CDs along the hallway for days to come…

It never ceased to amaze me how Mauricio's rage paralleled Mrs. Bromley's outbursts. When enraged over something that I supposedly have done wrong, my husband used to isolate himself in our bedroom, staring at the ceiling. He would tell the maids at home and the staff at his office that he was ill and was not to be disturbed. I moved to the guestroom because I didn't want to share a bed with a madman; everything was put on hold until I moved back and said I was sorry.

Now Mrs. Bromley's passive reaction made me wonder if she too was trying to manipulate me. She might feel guilty for stomping on my CDs and now is using blackmail on me. Once again, as I had so many times in my life, suppressed my own feelings and ran to Mrs. Bromley's room to attend to her needs. I thought I had escaped my destiny, but I was caught in its net again. Mrs. Bromley treated me like my husband did, therefore reminding me of him all the time.

To my dismay, Meri didn't return the following Saturday. Jane contacted an agency and hired a part-time helper, making it clear they were not to send an African American woman, in order to avoid an embarrassing situation due to Mrs. Bromley's prejudice. I took advantage of every opportunity to prepare Mrs. Bromley for the new woman who would take care of her on Saturdays.

"Mrs. Bromley, we're looking for a nice woman to fill in for me on my day off."

She raised her eyebrows. "I beg your pardon?"

"You know I need Saturdays off."

"No, I don't, and I don't care. You're not leaving me alone."

"That's precisely what I'm trying to explain. A woman will stay with you while I'm gone."

"Can you trust the woman? Is she smart? Is she clever?"

I chuckled, amused at her silly concerns. "She's been highly recommended," I said, anticipating her reaction.

"Recommended by whom?"

"Jane called an agency. The woman is coming tomorrow for an interview. And yes, we can trust her."

"Is she smart? Is she intelligent?" she insisted. "Does she have a nice personality?"

"Intelligent or not, what do you care? She'll take good care of you, and that's what matters."

"Your lack of social manners amazes me."

I was on the brink of saying *What the hell do social manners have to do with this?* Instead I said, "I'm sorry if I don't meet your high standards, but I'm here to take care of you, and that's what I do to the best of my ability."

She smiled. "Your highness, I only wanted to know if the woman is smart."

I hesitated before saying, "How would I know that? I haven't met her."

"All this time wasted babbling, when you could have said that you don't know. You should have admitted that from the beginning."

I didn't like to admit it, but she was right.

On Friday, the woman from the agency came for an interview. We were watching television when the front doorbell rang. Bowdie barked and ran to the door.

Mrs. Bromley rose from her chair. "Bowdie is acting up. Are we expecting company? They're too late for tea, so get rid of them."

"It must be the lady replacing Meri."

"Meri? Who's Meri?"

The bell rang again. Mrs. Bromley called Bowdie. "Easy, baby girl. Stop barking! And you, Lolita, open the door."

In an attempt to further prepare her, I said, "You're going to meet the lady who will take my place on Saturdays."

"I don't know what you're talking about. Just open the bloody door."

I opened the door and was surprised to see a heavyset black woman. I didn't know what to do. Finally I managed to say, "Come in, please."

Mrs. Bromley came up behind me. "Don't ask her in," she said. "We don't know who that woman is."

"Don't worry, Mrs. Bromley, we're expecting her," I said. Then, to the woman, "I'm afraid there's been a mistake. Perhaps the agency sent you in place of Gladys?"

"Ma'am, I am Gladys."

I didn't want to hurt her feelings, but I was upset that the agency hadn't complied with Jane's request.

"Please come in the living room," I said, smiling.

"Thank you, ma'am."

Gladys walked over to the couch and took a seat. Mrs. Bromley's icy-blue eyes were scrutinizing the woman. No one spoke. The silence weighed tons. I felt clumsy not finding an appropriate way to break the ice. I wished Mrs. Bromley would say something, but she seemed to have lost her tongue.

Finally Gladys spoke. "I'll be proud to take care of you, ma'am," she addressed Mrs. Bromley. "You look so pretty and dignified."

"I don't know what you're talking about," Mrs. Bromley blurted.

The woman giggled. "Your caregiver is off tomorrow, and I'll be happy to keep you company."

"You're absolutely wrong. If Lolita leaves me with you, she better stay away from this house."

"You don't like me, ma'am?" Gladys asked.

"Of course not."

"What is it you have against me, ma'am?"

"You do not want to know the answer." Mrs. Bromley said defiantly.

"I grow on people, ma'am. At first they don't like me much, and then they can't live without me. Give me a little time, please, ma'am."

"Stop ma'aming me!" Mrs. Bromley shouted.

Words failed me, but finally I was able to say, "I'm sorry, Gladys, it's impossible to reason with her. It's nothing personal; she's like that with me too. I'm very embarrassed."

Gladys got up, slowly. "It's a pity you ain't gonna find out how good I can take care of you. You should've given me a try," she said, with a sad smile.

I wanted to avoid looking Gladys in the eyes, but I gathered courage and took her hand. "Don't take it personally. She's sick, and a very difficult person to get along with."

"Oh, yeah, sick and also very bitter." She smiled at me, and I noticed tears rolling down her cheeks. "Don't you worry, ma'am," she said, wiping away her tears. "It's okay. There's a lot of other white folks that's fond of me."

"I'm fond of you already," I said truthfully.

"Lord bless you," Gladys said and left.

"Are you satisfied?" I asked, going back into the room. "Are you proud of the way you treated that poor woman?"

"How dare you lecture me? Your audacity amazes me."

"I think what amazes you is my compassion for people and your lack of it. You should treat human beings the way you'd like to be treated."

"Start by respecting my rights. Why did you bring a black person into my house in the first place? You should have known better."

I counted to ten and sat quietly as we watched television. Gladys's tears were embedded in my mind, breaking my heart. I wanted to give the person at the agency a piece of my mind, but the assurance that Jane would set them straight made me feel better.

24

Pine-Sol

With Meri out of the picture, I was determined to find a Saturday replacement for Mrs. Bromley. I tried to convince Jane to cover for me, but she didn't want to spend any more time than necessary with Mrs. Bromley.

After several weeks of missing my writers' group, I decided to discuss my dilemma with Meri again. We met for coffee at a sidewalk café, after my Spanish class one Wednesday afternoon. After exchanging pleasantries, it didn't take long for me to broach the topic of Mrs. Bromley.

I told Meri what experience had taught me: trying to reason with Mrs. Bromley was the wrong way to approach her. It saddened me that Meri didn't share my point of view.

"Okay, Lolita, she may be sick, but I think she gets away with everything because we give in to her too easily. If she's like a child, as you say, then we need to be more firm with her."

"Children have growing, fresh brains that we can mold. Mrs. Bromley's mind is dysfunctional and is deteriorating rapidly. Even though she acts like a child, we need to treat her like the sick person she is."

"Yes," Meri said to the waitress in front of us. "We'd like two cappuccinos, please."

"You know, Meri," I continued, "in the beginning, I used to cry a lot and I wanted to quit almost every day. I'm glad I didn't because I control the situation now. I let her rave and rant, and once she lets off steam, she calms down by herself. I don't have unbearable situations anymore."

"Lolita, we're different. I can't cope with this situation. I'm afraid I have a deep psychological problem. My mother used to blackmail me by pretending to be sick all the time. She made my life miserable by forcing me to cater to her every whim. When I see Mrs. Bromley going through one of her tantrums, my mother comes to mind." Meri paused for a moment. She seemed troubled. "I'll be right back," she said. "I'm going to powder my nose."

Meri's confession left me concerned. I couldn't in good conscience insist that she take care of Mrs. Bromley when doing so brought back such painful memories. The same thing was true for Jane. Due to the animosity between them, any little thing could ignite violence. This awareness came to spoil everything, because if Mrs. Bromley had already become violent with Meri, next time it could be worse. If Jane had slapped Mrs. Bromley and left her with bruises, then next time…*On the other hand, she is not my family and I am not Mother Theresa. As it is, I no longer have a life away from Mrs. Bromley. I'm doing what not even her own family is willing to do. I'm only asking for a few hours per week. I need time for myself or I'll go mad. I should stop worrying and keep insisting with Meri.*

Meri came back from the bathroom at the same time our cappuccinos arrived.

"Meri," I said, "regarding what you just told me about your mother, I'm sorry she traumatized you that way."

"And you don't know the half of it. She was cruel. I still have scars on my knees—one of her ways of punishment was to have me kneel on bottle caps for hours."

I placed my hand on hers. "I'm sorry, my friend. It's hard to believe that your own mother did such cruel things to you."

"I forgave her but I can't forget. My childhood was a nightmare. I don't remember a good thing about her. I'm just full of resentment."

I was sorry for Meri, but I didn't know how to console her.

"Meri, let's go back to Mrs. Bromley. I won't pretend not to have my own agenda when trying to convince you to help me with her, but I also believe that in order for you, as a victim of abuse, to get over it and go on with your life, you need to confront and forgive the abuser. You need to overcome the trauma your mother created, and since she's no longer with us, see Mrs. Bromley as you would your mother. Forgive and forget both of them. Start a new life with an open mind. Do what I do: I cover my senses with soap so offenses slid."

"It's not the same. I think I could get past all the craziness if she weren't such a snobbish and ungrateful bitch. She brings the worst in me." Meri paused for a moment and went on, "The thing is that I'm very compassionate with humble people and I'll do anything for them. With Mrs. Bromley, it is different. She's snobbish and ungrateful, and that builds a barrier between us. She's got the money to buy whatever she wants. Let the family find somebody else to replace you, but not me."

"Jane called an agency and they sent over a nice black lady, but you know how Mrs. Bromley is. It didn't work."

"That's what I mean—she's spoiled rotten. If she didn't want a black person, you should have given her an ultimatum. She either accepts the woman or stays by herself. That might shake her into becoming less picky. It's worth a try, don't you think?"

"Uh, it won't work, either," I said.

Meri sighed. "I know. She's prejudiced and too set in her ways. But, Lolita, that shouldn't be your problem. I myself rather care for an old, sweet woman for free than for Mrs. Bromley with all her money."

"Be realistic Meri. No sweet old woman will pay like Mrs. Bromley does, and you know it."

"Good pay? What about peace of mind? I wouldn't trade my health for all the money in the world."

"Don't be so stubborn, Meri. It's only once a week. Admit it, you need the money as much as I do. Please, replace me on Saturdays. I miss my writers' group so much." Meri looked at me, and I read sympathy in her eyes. "I'll return right after the meeting," I continued. "That way you can leave sooner, and I'll even give you more money."

Meri patted my hand. "You didn't hear me. You didn't get my point. I don't care about money. That woman makes me feel like a beggar, like she's saving my life. If I felt needed and appreciated, I'd put up with almost anything."

"Well, I need you. I appreciate you, and I'll be in your debt for the rest of my life if you come back to work on Saturdays."

She didn't answer right away. I knew she was right. Mrs. Bromley never showed appreciation for what we did for her; rather, she took it for granted that if she paid, she had the right to demand.

"I'm going to tell you how she mistreated me," Meri said after a while.

"Is there more than what I already know?"

"I kept most of it to myself, but I'll tell you something that happened recently." She hesitated. "She struck me with a cane."

I was horrified, but when Meri chuckled, I suspected it couldn't have been that serious. "How did it happen?"

"Well, one time she snuck out of the house, and I found her across the street in her panties and nothing else, talking with a sour-faced guy. She asked him out, and he said no, but she ignored his refusal. I was so embarrassed.

"She called him Robert and told him she'd be back in a tick and something about him being her guest. Then he told her he wasn't Robert and that if she didn't get dressed he'd call the police."

I found Meri's story hard to believe, but with Mrs. Bromley, anything was possible. I wondered why Mrs. Bromley didn't behave that way around me. Could it be because I never let her out of my sight, and never contradicted her unless absolutely necessary?

"I'm telling you, Lolita," Meri continued, "if looks could kill, the guy would have killed us. He did call the police, but we were gone before the patrol car arrived."

"But Meri, what was she doing outside in the first place? Why naked? How come you didn't notice when she went out?"

"I thought I could watch TV in my room while she napped."

"People with Alzheimer's are like babies." I tried not to sound judgmental, but I didn't like what I was hearing. "You can let them out of your mind, but never out of your sight." Meri looked worried, but I wanted to know why Mrs. Bromley had hit her, and although afraid of the answer, I still asked, "Now, what happened with the cane?"

"Well, on the way back to the house, I chided her. She mimicked everything I said and stuck her tongue out. I angrily screamed, 'Don't you dare do that to me!' She grabbed a cane from the stand, and I ran away, but she caught up with me and struck me several times. I admit she didn't use all her strength—It seemed like she wanted to scare me more than to hurt me, but she wasn't playing either, because she looked mad as hell."

It was obvious that Jane and Meri triggered a violent streak in Mrs. Bromley. And to think that Saturdays used to go so well in the beginning. Meri had given Mrs. Bromley all her attention; what a pity that Meri had run out of patience. Also, it seemed the illness was advancing and Mrs. Bromley was going through mood swings more often.

"Jane wanted to put a chain at the top of the door, so Mrs. Bromley couldn't get out of the house without being heard," I told this to Meri because I wanted her to be up to date on what was going on with Mrs. Bromley. "But I knew that if she found herself locked in, it would provoke a violent outburst, so I suggested a bell instead, that way we'd know every time she opened the front door."

"I think the lock is better and safer," Meri said.

"I disagree, and let me tell you why. Last week, when I took her to the hairdresser, Linda said it was going to take close to three hours. I didn't want to sit around and wait that long, so I decided to get a perm too. I should have anticipated that something could go wrong."

"Did you really ask for a perm?"

"Yes."

"*Ay, chihuahua*, how could you?"

"I know I was foolish. Have you noticed how paranoid she gets when we do something personal on her time? When she saw the hairdresser working on me, she didn't want her nails or feet done, so she paid her bill and told the girl to call a taxi. I begged Mrs. Bromley to wait just a few minutes while Linda took the rollers off. She said her principles would not allow her to wait for me when we were on her time. Linda locked the door so she could finish my perm. Mrs. Bromley tried to open it, and when she couldn't, she got hysterical and began screaming and banging on the door. Linda had to open it, and Mrs. Bromley left. I ran out to look for her. I went into the nearby stores and supermarket, but nobody had seen her."

"*Caramba*, what did you do next?"

"I went back to the beauty salon and the hairdresser called a couple of taxi stands to find out if any driver had picked up an old lady walking by herself around the vicinity, but no luck. I tried to be calm as Linda took my rollers out, but inside I was frantic and didn't know what I would say to the family." I paused and then asked Meri, "Do you remember when I left her alone to go to church? Mr. Williams was nice about it then, but I doubt he'd be that understanding a second time. Before calling the police, I decided to go to her house to make the necessary calls from there. When I arrived I couldn't believe it when I found her sitting in the living room."

"Unbelievable! How did she get there?"

"I don't know, but I was so relieved to see that she was safe that I hugged her. As usual, she pushed me away. When I questioned her about how she had gotten home, she said that she didn't remember."

"What if she remembers and tells her family?"

"I don't know. But it's going to haunt me all my life as to how she got home."

We continued to talk a long time. I tried everything I knew to persuade Meri to replace me on Saturdays. As a last resort, I appealed to her sensitivity. I knew material things would never influence her, so I asked in the name of our friendship to do it for me. I told her the truth, that I needed this job desperately, but if I continued at this pace I was going to go mad.

Finally, Meri took pity on me and said she'd work half a day on Saturdays, making it clear that it was only to help me and that I was to be back as soon as the meetings were over.

From then on, Saturdays went well. Little by little, I forgot our arrangement about getting back right after the meetings. I extended my stay longer each Saturday, attending the group luncheons. I owed one to Meri, because she was very understanding. One Saturday, I explained to her that I needed the whole day off and that I was going to get back very late because I was hosting a Mexican party at my house.

I usually began to enjoy my parties from the moment of their conception. I always loved live music and shows in my fiestas, so I hired a band of mariachis, and with the help of other members of the singles' club we prepared the grounds for the party. We had balloons and all kinds of Mexican decorations: sombreros, zarapes, maracas, piñatas, colorful masks, and bark paintings. The tablecloths and napkins were of typical bright colors. I had most of the food catered by a restaurant in Tampa.

I had CDs and cassettes playing my favorite music all day long while preparing for the fiesta. Memories invaded me, and I began to recall many past parties.

I was supposed to be the hostess in our mansion in Mexico, but I was just another ornament. Mauricio showed off his house and his young beautiful wife, loaded with jewelry. I was brainwashed to believe that all that glitter was synonymous with happiness. Those were parties without soul…empty. The guests were businesspeople, industrialists, and politicians, and the warmth that friends bring just wasn't there. That was in Mexico, where I was merely my husband's shadow. But my parties in this other part of the world were very different. My spirit was there, and I was the head of the show. I did the shopping, the cleaning, and some of the cooking; I made all of the necessary arrangements, which made me feel accomplished. At last, I had found my voice. I didn't play the hostess; I *was* the hostess. My soul and my mind were there. Fulfillment came from the inside out, and once on the surface, it translated into happiness. I shared those times with friends who were interested in having a good time, not in concocting future earnings. And though the guests at my parties in Florida were well-to-do people, they came to the party to forget business and live the moment—and that made all the difference.

The time to get ready for the party arrived, and I raced up the steps leading to my bedroom, ready to make my best effort and get dressed to impress. I wore a black diaphanous dress with hand-painted pink and purple flowers. Since I didn't have time to go to the beauty salon, I let my hair drape over my shoulders. I was satisfied with the results. I felt confident and in the best mood to enjoy my party. This was a party afforded by my own efforts. Could this be called independence?

The mariachis played happy music like "Cielito Lindo" and "Rancho Grande," the music that reminded me of Tito Guizar and of my youth. My guests knew some of the words, so we all sang along with the band.

But...In the midst of dinner, I received a call from Meri. She sounded alarmed.

"Can you come immediately?"

"I can't leave my guests. What's wrong?"

"I just called 911."

"What? Why?" I asked, as the blood drained from my face.

"She drank Pine-Sol."

"What?"

"I need to go. The ambulance is here," she said, and hung up.

"Call me from the hospital!" I cried out too late, Meri wasn't there anymore.

Gloom replaced the exuberant happiness that had filled me a second before. I explained to Jane Olson, the president of the club, what had happened, to take over and to continue with the party.

I sped my way to Mrs. Bromley's. As I opened the door, I felt emptiness in my heart and a knot in my stomach. I felt spent. No one but Bowdie was there. I wanted to ask it what had happened, but she couldn't tell me. My heart sank when I saw the image of Mrs. Bromley dying.

I wondered how she had gotten hold of the Pine-Sol and how much she had drank. How serious was it? I wanted to run to her side and make sure she was going to be all right. *Please, God*, I prayed, *spare her.*

I looked at Bowdie. I knew from her inquisitive gaze that she wanted to know how Mrs. Bromley was doing as much as I did. The poor thing wanted to know why she had been left alone after so much commotion. Her eyes reflected emptiness, and she looked so sad. It dawned on me how much I had grown to care for the little dog. Her distress awoke my real feelings. I took her in my arms, ignoring my fine dress, and began to use the same lingo Mrs. Bromley used. I told Bowdie not to worry, because her mother would be home soon, and in the meantime, Mama Lolita would be right here next to her.

"Yes, Bowdie, don't worry! My treasure, I love you."

Was that me talking? Was I feeling the impulse to kiss a dog? Yes, I felt like holding the little furry thing against my heart and kissing her until her sadness vanished away and life came back into her listless eyes. Yes, love must be blind. I wanted to make Bowdie happy and take her pain away as you do with a defenseless child. Quite the contrast from the vision I once held of a filthy animal. Now I understood the adoration that many people have for their pets.

After an hour of anxious waiting, I called Jane and left a message on her machine, then I called Mr. Williams's cell phone and left another message. Finally, he called back with some news. Meri had been cleaning, he explained, and left the Pine-Sol on the counter. Mrs. Bromley drank the Pine-Sol mistaking it for juice. Meri called an ambulance and took her to the emergency room because she refused to ride in Meri's car. The paramedics had to forcibly strap her to a wheelchair. In the hospital she had been unruly. They had tied her hands and feet while waiting for Mr. Williams. Finally he got there and signed a release.

Since he had to go back to a family reunion, Jane had to stay until a doctor pumped her stomach. Thankfully, Mr. Williams gave me the phone number and the name of the hospital.

I called immediately, and Meri explained that Jane had just left. Mrs. Bromley was recuperating, and as soon as she was better, they'd be back home.

"Meri, what was a bottle of Pine-Sol doing on the counter?" I asked.

"I took it out to clean the kitchen."

"We don't have to clean anything. Beside, that kitchen is immaculate."

"I like to clean, and since I got bored, I looked for something to do."

"When you are at her house, you only have to take care of her," I said bluntly. I couldn't believe that Meri had done that, when we were there solely to look after Mrs. Bromley.

When they arrived way past midnight, they found Bowdie and me sleeping on my bed.

Although Meri was exhausted, she refused to stay overnight.

"I feel sick. I can't bear to hear another word out of her mouth," Meri said despondently. Then she said, with an edge of irony, "Well, I never thought I was going to see you sleeping so comfortably with a dog in your arms. I hope you enjoy your newfound family."

Meri left and I took Bowdie to Mrs. Bromley's bedroom.

25

The End?

I had never felt the need to turn on the intercom, but that night I did. I heard Mrs. Bromley moaning and mumbling. I checked on her several times, but she was always asleep, with Bowdie by her side.

The following day, she didn't get out of bed as usual. I found her struggling to go to the bathroom, so I helped her back to bed and sat nearby with a book.

"That's what they did to me," she said, staring at her arm.

"What did they do to you?"

"Those monsters. They tried to kill me. They put me in jail." She looked like she was going to cry. "*Mon Dieu*, Robert, don't leave me alone. Put me out of this misery. Where are you, my Robert?"

"Mrs. Bromley," I said, hoping to comfort her, "I'm here with you. Don't be afraid."

"There's nothing you can do to save me from them."

"Who are *them*, dear?"

"My family, who else? They want to commit me, but I don't want to leave my house."

"Please, don't think like that. Your family is all you have, and they love you. They care for you."

"Putting me away is a clever way to get to my money," she whispered.

"Mr. Williams and Jane were here this morning, but you were sleeping. They also have been calling during the day to find out about your progress." I altered the truth. "They are very concerned."

"Before I am gone, those vultures will divest me of all my possessions."

My poor Mrs. Bromley, since the awful experience from the Pine-Sol incident she seemed hunted and confused. *How can I bring her back from those dreadful memories?*

I ran my fingers through her hair. "I wish you could see the pretty waves in your hair," I said. "You have beautiful curls at the end."

"That's the only thing left from the beauty I once possessed," she lamented.

I was happy to divert her attention.

"Well," I continued, "not only that, but your teeth. How many people can keep their own teeth and their own hair at your age?"

"How old am I?"

"You're ninety-one."

"You're lying!"

I decided to call Jane to explain her situation. She advised me not to worry, and said Mrs. Bromley's reaction was normal after what she had gone through in the hospital.

"I made an appointment to take her to the doctor on Wednesday," she said.

"I'd be more than happy to take her tomorrow," I said. "I don't think we should wait."

"There's no need to be concerned, but thank you for offering."

"But Jane, it's better to prevent—"

"Lolita," she interrupted. "I appreciate your interest, but I'll take her on Wednesday."

I had no other choice but to mind my own business.

By Tuesday, I was really worried. It was pitiful to see Mrs. Bromley's health deteriorating so rapidly. Three days earlier she had been full of energy, and now she was drained and lifeless. She started to babble, which concerned me because I couldn't tell if she was asking for something.

The shock of finding herself tied to a bed, surrounded by tubes and nurses, must have been devastating. I never imagined that Mrs. Bromley's sudden and rapid deterioration would hit me so hard and wondered how Jane could be so detached from her mother-in-law's condition.

The thought that no one was exempt from Alzheimer's terrorized me. Usually every time I forgot something, I blamed it on distraction, but now I feared that my forgetfulness could be a prelude to the treacherous illness. In the face of this reality, I reaffirmed my pledge to treat her with the same respect I'd like to have if destiny placed me in a similar situation, but with one big exception: I wouldn't have Mrs. Bromley's luxury of one-on-one care. What happened to people with no money and no insurance?

I had always believed that you reap what you sow. In light of that, I asked God for patience and the wisdom to handle Mrs. Bromley's situation without failing in the process. It was beneficial for me to often reaffirm my good intentions. I promised to devote my life to her for as long as she needed me.

When I had started working for Mrs. Bromley, she was energetic and witty. Despite her dementia, her will was so strong that I thought no one could ever bend or break it. I had always felt her presence, because her strong personality filled the room. At first, her overpowering personality annoyed me. Now I longed to have it back.

I continually leaned forward, trying to make out her words, or at least read her thoughts. I prayed.

I rejoiced when she finally got out of bed and walked around the house, leaning against the walls to support herself. I offered my help, but she refused it. To my dismay, she fell down and I couldn't help her to get up. She crawled to a chair, and then I helped her to get up and back to bed.

"Are you cold, Lolita?" she asked, and then giggled like a little girl.

"I'm okay, thanks."

"Here, this will help to warm you." She handed me two hairpins. "I'm sure this will keep you warm."

I took the pins from her hand. "Thank you, Mrs. Bromley," I said, holding back tears. "It's very kind of you."

"Haven't I always been kind?" she asked.

Drawn on an impulse I wanted to hug her, so I threw my arms around her shoulders. She shoved me away softly with shaking hands, as if she weren't sure whether she wanted to be embraced. Maybe that was a cultural thing. On the other hand I thought the balsamic effect of touching was universal and very human. I'll wait. A day will come when she'll search for refuge in my arms. People needed human touch to feel safe and wanted.

When I returned from my day off on Wednesday, Mrs. Bromley was back to her old self. Jane had taken her to a Chinese doctor for acupuncture to alleviate the pain in her shoulder, a treatment to which I was to take her twice a week.

"Lolita," Jane said as she was leaving, "when Betty saw the doctor, she told him that he was exactly what her doctor ordered. So don't worry." Jane laughed and concluded, "We'll have Betty with us for a while yet."

On Friday, I took Mrs. Bromley to her second acupuncture appointment. "Where are we going that Bowdie can't come?" she asked.

"You have an appointment with a very handsome doctor."

"What handsome doctor? Be specific."

"The one Jane took you to last Wednesday, the one you liked a lot."

"Did he like me?"

"I wasn't with you that day, but I'm sure he did."

"*Bon*. He'd better be good-looking."

When we arrived at the doctor's office, there were several people ahead of us, so we sat down and waited. Mrs. Bromley was getting impatient, and I was nervously expecting an outburst. I froze when she abruptly stood up and walked to the receptionist's desk.

"Is it your policy to keep patients waiting indefinitely?" she asked.

I jumped to my feet and joined her. "Mrs. Bromley, please," I whispered, "sit down and wait for your turn."

"You'd better keep out of this!" she shouted. "This young woman had better do something, or we are leaving."

I wanted to run to my refuge, the bathroom. Just then, a tall, handsome Caucasian doctor entered the waiting room.

"Good morning, Mrs. Bromley," he said pleasantly. "What a delight to see you again."

Mrs. Bromley turned to face him, and her impatience melted into a flirtatious smile. He escorted her to a connecting room across from the waiting parlor. With the door ajar, he handed her a robe.

"Put this on. I'll be right back," he said and walked away.

In a few moments, she opened the door and stood there, stark naked. I rushed to her. "Mrs. Bromley, put on the robe."

"Tell the doctor that I'm ready!" she said.

Oh, goodness, how embarrassing. The patients in the waiting room pretended to read, but they took in the scene out of the corner of their eyes. The receptionist hurriedly left the room and came back with the doctor.

"Mrs. Bromley, put on the robe," he said with a straight face, in a firm but kind voice. "Let your lady-friend help you."

"I prefer you to help me," Mrs. Bromley said, with a mischievous smile.

The doctor addressed me. "Please, will you see that she puts on the robe?"

Later on, the receptionist called Jane and scheduled after-hours appointments for the rest of her treatments.

The next morning, to my delight, Mrs. Bromley was on her best behavior. After breakfast, she placed her address book in my hand. "Lolita," she said, "look up Bill's address so we can go visit him. Don't bother to call."

"We need to call first," I said. "Remember? He's never home." "It doesn't matter; we'll go just the same. I bought his house, so I'm entitled to see it."

Bill was her old-time gay friend whom she often had me call. I also sent letters, but he never replied. On several occasions, she had wanted to visit "the person she trusted most in the world." Until now, I had been able to dodge driving her to Cocoa Beach. Now that my feelings for her had changed, it was more difficult not to please her. Still, it was a long drive, and I was sure Mr. Williams wouldn't approve of it.

"We'll visit him later."

"Now! Get Bowdie's towel and let's go. Bring some treats and water for her."

"It's too early. Let's call him first and make sure he's there." *If I could buy some time, maybe she'd forget.*

"No, let's go right now," she insisted.

"I need to go to the bathroom," I said.

"I don't know what's wrong with you. You spend your whole life in bathrooms. I'm sure a doctor can enlarge your bladder. Hurry up. I'll wait in the car."

This time my ploy didn't work. Now what would I do? There was no way I was going to drive her there. I had to comply with Jane and Mr. Williams's wishes.

"Hurry up Lolita. If you must go to the bathroom, don't take all day. We have a long trip ahead of us."

I pondered the situation and decided to take her to Sarasota instead. I enjoyed the drive across the Sunshine Skyway Bridge, and maybe the beautiful scenery would take her mind off Bill.

Mrs. Bromley was in the car with Bowdie by the time I got to the garage. I hoped she might have forgotten about Bill, so I said, "Okay, Mrs. Bromley, where to?"

"Do you take me for a fool, or are you just an idiot?"

"What are you talking about?"

"You might be stupid, but I'm not. Take me to Bill's once and for all."

"I'm sorry. You're right. For a moment, I forgot."

When we reached Sarasota, I tested her again. "We have arrived. Are you hungry? Should I look for a nice restaurant?" I was afraid of what I would hear.

"Are you really stupid?"

"Mrs. Bromley, it's not nice to insult me. You're hurting my feelings," I said.

"Then what do you think you're doing with mine? Taking me for an imbecile, an idiot, a dummy, or what?"

"I don't understand why you are so mad."

"You mean you don't know we are in Sarasota and not in Cocoa Beach?

"Oh? How do you know?" I asked, surprises that she knew where we were.

"I can read, you know. All the signs say Sarasota. We haven't reached Cocoa Beach yet."

Once more, I had underestimated this amazing woman. I gently squeezed her hand. "Oh, Mrs. Bromley, please forgive me. You're right. I'll ask the way to Cocoa Beach at a gas station. I'm very sorry."

She pulled her hand away. "*Bon.* Don't waste any more time here. Let's just go."

I drove in silence, listening to her talk to Bowdie about how stupid Lolita was. I stopped at a Chevron station and looked around until I saw a distinguished, middle-aged man. I rolled down the window on Mrs. Bromley's side, so she could hear the conversation and enjoy his closeness.

"May I help you?" he asked.

She smiled the smile she saved for men. "Be an angel and tell my companion how to get to Cocoa Beach."

"My dear ladies, you're very far away. Cocoa Beach is south of Orlando."

"How long will it take?" she asked, still smiling.

"Maybe three or four hours from here."

At that moment, I expected her insults to spew out of her mouth, but she was too busy savoring the conversation with him to waste her time with reprimands.

"Please, Mrs. Bromley, forgive me. I've made such a big mistake."

"You didn't do it on purpose. Get a paper and pen, and this handsome gentleman will give you directions on how to get to Bill's house."

Although I didn't need any explication, I allowed the man to give me directions, so Mrs. Bromley could be in his presence a little longer. I couldn't keep pretending that I didn't understand. He was very patient, repeating the directions more than enough times to be understood.

I finally said, "Thanks a million. I think I know how to get there now."

"I should think so," Mrs. Bromley said. She turned to the man. "I can't tell you how much I appreciated your help. Now, will you be kind enough to have lunch with us?"

"Thank you," he said, "but my wife is waiting for me."

"Oh, well," Mrs. Bromley insisted, "perhaps you could call her and—"

I quickly interrupted, "Thank you, sir. You've done your good deed for the day. Thanks again."

"Lolita," she said as we drove out of the gas station, "why didn't you grab that handsome man? You should have asked him out."

"He's married," I replied. "You heard him. His wife is waiting for him."

"Oh, Lolita, that was just an excuse to an older woman. Maybe if you had asked, he would have accepted."

"Mrs. Bromley, where I come from, we don't ask men out, specially if they're married and young enough to be your sons."

"Well," she proclaimed, "I'm sure you have an overpopulation of old maids in your country."

I laughed. "Do you want to stop at a restaurant?"

"I'm not hungry," she replied, "but Bowdie and I need to tinkle."

I drove north toward St. Pete Beach. On the way, I stopped at a McDonald's overlooking the bay. I helped her out of the car and put the leash on Bowdie...

"Mrs. Bromley, if you like, you can sit here and wait while Bowdie does her business. Then we'll go to the bathroom inside the restaurant."

"Good thinking, Lolita. The weather is pleasant, so I'll watch the seagulls while you take care of my baby. She's been so patient."

I walked Bowdie near the seawall. Strangely enough, I found myself scrutinizing what the dog was about to do. Was she doing number two? How many? What size? Did it come out easily?

Although I used to hate it, lately I had voluntarily updated Mrs. Bromley on Bowdie's bowel movements. If Bowdie struggled to produce results, I would dispense a teaspoon of mineral oil in her food. How funny. I was concerned because the dog was constipated, but why hadn't I given such a personal attention to my children when they were growing up? I had left the job to the nannies. I realized now that there was a certain sense of fulfillment and accomplishment when you take care of things instead of having others do things for you. I felt strangely satisfied with the new me, though very sorry I couldn't go back to the past and do things differently.

As I walked Bowdie, I kept an eye on Mrs. Bromley. When I saw her get up and go into the restaurant, I tossed the dog in the back of the car and ran inside.

She was sitting down and banging on the table.

"This is lousy service. I want a waitress!" she yelled.

"They don't have waitresses in MacDonald's," I said.

"What kind of a bloody restaurant is this?" She turned to a man who was carrying his tray and asked, "Will you please bring me a glass of wine?"

The man looked at her and kept walking. She jumped up and grabbed his shirt. "I am talking to you, young man. Bring me a glass of rosé."

"I don't work here," the man said, and pulled away from her grasp.

"Then why are you carrying that tray?" she shouted after him. She turned to me. "You certainly did an extraordinary job choosing this restaurant."

As people stared at us, I tried to calm her down. "Mrs. Bromley, we only came here to use the facilities. This is a fast-food restaurant."

"I don't see any fast action here. On the contrary, they are really slow."

"We need to go." I said.

"I haven't tinkled yet."

"Okay, go in that door. I'll be right here when you're done."

"Don't you dare move from here."

When I saw her coming out of the ladies' room, I rushed over. "We can leave now, Mrs. Bromley."

"I demand attention. I want to eat here, and I will."

"Before we order, we have to take care of Bowdie. She's outside and not on a leash. It's very hot outside," I exaggerated.

"*Mon Dieu*! My baby! Hurry up before she suffocates or someone kills her. Go."

We went outside, and she looked around. "Where's my baby?" she cried out. "Lolita, you're responsible for this! I'll kill you if I don't find Bowdie."

"She's in the car; don't worry."

"Why did you tell me she was loose?" she asked angrily.

"I'm sorry. I told you she was outside the restaurant. I forgot to mention she was in the car."

"You shouldn't be taking care of my treasure if you're suffering from memory loss."

She never ceased to amaze me. "Yes, Mrs. Bromley," I said. "You're right."

We drove north to St. Pete Beach. Just when I thought Bill was out of her mind, she started again.

"Lolita, what's wrong with you? We're going to Cocoa Beach."

"The man told us that Cocoa Beach was south of Orlando, and Orlando is north so we have to go back past St. Pete Beach. Don't worry; now we're on the right track."

"You're not allowed to make another mistake. Be careful now."

I hoped that by the time we stopped to eat, the idea of visiting Bill would be out of her mind.

While she talked to the dog, I prayed. After we drove over the Skyway Bridge, I stopped at the Leverocks restaurant on 34th Street.

Luckily after a few drinks, she forgot about Cocoa Beach.

That night, while getting ready for bed, I remembered the days when my children were growing up with governesses and nannies. I never knew when they were constipated or if they were having problems, unless they made me aware of it.

How I longed for the opportunity to go back in time and do things differently. My children's childhood was gone forever, and I never got the chance to participate in their experiences. Mauricio had instilled low self-esteem in me, and he had made it clear that I wasn't the mother he wanted for his children. The governess knew many languages, was sophisticated and familiar with the glitter of high society. I felt insignificant. I was resentful that Mauricio hadn't thought of the consequences before he married me.

I was a dreamer from a middle-class part of Havana, swept off my feet by a debonair, worldly man. He had solved my family's financial problems and provided me with a comfortable future. Mauricio had given me luxuries and trips abroad that before were only fantasies for me.

I wanted to further my education, but he was against it. He knew that by denying me knowledge, he reinforced the path to my slavery. I was young and easily deceived then, so I blindly followed his arbitrary rules, unaware that what he really wanted was to divest me of the right to be myself. I allowed him to usurp my identity.

By Mauricio's standards, my humble upbringing hindered my ability to teach my children class and good manners; therefore, he trusted them to the governess.

In hindsight, it was clear to me that he had overlooked my lack of formal education because it helped to keep me from rebelling and assured him ownership. He had considered me his beautiful trophy wife, whom he draped in gold and diamonds to show off to his business associates. I was a costly ornament to feed his ego. My intellect was in his way.

Now I realized that I had exchanged a humble life for a purposeless wealthy one. I hated myself for having wasted my time and energy in superficial matters, for ignoring my roots, and for burying my values under a blanket of empty wealth.

26

Beloved Bowdie

As time passed by, everything remained about the same, with its usual ups and downs. The only thing that changed was my attitude. Finally I became immune to Mrs. Bromley's insults and tantrums. I was amazed at how the same behavior that once had hurt me now left my spirit unscathed. I was sorry it hadn't worked that way during my marriage.

My husband's contempt had never ceased to crush me. It still hurt. The change in my attitude placed me in a more comfortable position. Now I belonged to the Bromley's household. I turned over my heart to her, and my intuition told me she felt the same way. But in the midst of my change of heart, an offer came along to challenge my peace of mind: a full-time job as a companion to a writer who had been partly paralyzed due to a car accident.

On the night I received the offer, I couldn't sleep, I struggled against the temptation to accept such an ideal opportunity. The job was closer to my house, with a better salary and a one-in-a-million chance to take care of an author. She might be willing to teach me creative writing on a one-on-one basis, furthermore, there was the possibility of escorting her to conferences and seminars in addition to meeting other writers. That was enough to entice me.

I was torn thinking it would be inconsiderate on my part to leave Mrs. Bromley, knowing how hard it would be to find a person willing to put up with her. I thought Mr. Williams would probably have no other alternative but to place her in a nursing home, where she'd be sedated all the time.

I spent hours pondering about the advantages and disadvantages of this new opportunity. My dream was that if I learned to write well, I could make it in the literary world; but if I left Mrs. Bromley and something happened to her, I wouldn't be able to enjoy my success. The guilt would stay with me forever. I asked my guardian angel to help me make the right decision. I meditated and prayed for guidance, for a sign showing me the way. I tried to divert my attention in different directions, but to no avail. I ended up going back to consider my situation. I had grown to love Mrs. Bromley, and in moments of lucidity, she seemed to love me. The truth was that she totally relied on me; in fact, the whole family did. I felt my place was with her, but I worried, because this opportunity wasn't going to cross my path again. I envisioned myself writing a great novel. I reflected on the chances this country offered. The American Dream could be mine. The break was there for me to take, and I decided to take it.

Once I made up my mind to take the new job, I stood firm, focused on my future as a writer. I was going to write about Mrs. Bromley's struggle with Alzheimer's. Now the problem was how to break the news to Mr. Williams. Although the new job was to start right away, I felt I owed Mrs. Bromley at least two weeks' notice for her family to find a replacement. So I went to visit Mr. Williams.

As always, he welcomed me with a friendly smile. He sat across from me in the living room couch, and I began to wring my hands. I couldn't find the right words to convey my decision, but suddenly it just came out.

"I'm sorry to tell you this, but I'm leaving in two weeks because an opportunity has come my way, which I can't turn down."

His smile froze.

I felt terrible. I wasn't prepared for his response.

"You lasted longer than I ever expected," he said with a slight smile. "Have you finally given up on my grandmother?"

"Nothing of the sort," I said quickly, "I love her, and that's why I hate having to leave."

Apparently, he wasn't prepared for my answer either.

"Then I don't understand you, Lolita. I was always on your side and never paid attention to her complaints." He stood and shook his head. "So you love her, but you're leaving. Why? Do you want more money? Is that it? How much more do you want?"

I rose from the couch. "I appreciate your offer Mr. Williams, but money isn't the issue." I paused and cleared my throat. "I love to write, and I have an opportunity to be a companion to a successful author. To me, that's the chance of a lifetime. Can you please try to understand?"

He scratched his chin. "I'm certainly willing to offer you more money, but I can't make a writer out of my grandmother. We're going to miss you more than words can say, but I understand."

"Oh Mr. Williams, I'm so sorry, thank you!" I said relieved, but contrite at the same time.

"I hope I can find a person—"

"I'll help you," I cut in. "I'll talk to my Spanish friends. Maybe we can find the right person. I'll help you in any way possible."

We agreed. His understanding and kindness made my decision ever more painful. I almost wished this new job had never come along.

We told Mrs. Bromley that I was going to stay with my family in Mexico. She became agitated and angry, shouting at me repeatedly, "I don't know what you're going to do in a third-world country!"

"My family is there, and I have to go," I lied.

I asked all my friends but I couldn't find any that spoke enough English to take over my job with Mrs. Bromley. The trial period to choose my replacement began. For days, we interviewed women who answered our ad. None of them suited Mrs. Bromley.

One particular afternoon, we interviewed a woman named Cindy. When it was over, Cindy didn't make any attempt to leave. I stood up and said, "Thank you for coming. We'll let you know."

She didn't take the hint and remained seated.

"Lolita," Mrs. Bromley said harshly, "it is time to take Bowdie to the park. Tell this person to leave."

"Mrs. Bromley, please!"

Cindy leapt to her feet.

"Mrs. Bromley, please, don't be mean. You don't need to be rude."

I recalled my first scary interview in this house and Mrs. Bromley's rudeness.

"Thank you for your time," Cindy said. "And please, don't call me. I'm not interested in the job."

Embarrassed, I walked her to the door. "I'm sorry. Excuse her, please."

"Don't worry about it," she replied. "I'm glad I found out what I would have to put up with ahead of time. Good evening."

I regretted the loss of another prospect. I liked Cindy, and my hopes had risen for a moment.

"Lolita, don't waste time," Mrs. Bromley said as she took Bowdie outside. "Look for the leash, and we'll wait in the yard."

I went to her bedroom and grabbed the leash. As I reached the front door, I had a premonition that something terrible was about to happen. Then I heard screeching tires and a loud thump. Mrs. Bromley was crying frantically. I rushed outside and saw Bowdie lying on the ground. I went numb. The driver jumped out of his car and picked up the limp Bowdie, but Mrs. Bromley snatched her away from him.

"Lolita, bring a big towel!" she screamed. "Get the car! We've got to go for help!"

The driver was obviously distressed. "I've got a towel in my car. Please get in. We need to hurry." He turned to me. "We can't waste time. I'm taking them to the animal hospital in Pasadena. Follow us." He wrapped Bowdie in the towel, waited for Mrs. Bromley to get in, and then handed the dog to her.

I wondered how Bowdie got out. I assumed that Cindy must have left the gate open.

I left a message at Mr. Williams's office and sped toward the animal hospital. When I arrived there, the driver rushed over to me.

"I'm so sorry lady, It looks bad," he said. "Is there anything else I can do? At the very least, I'd like to pay the bill."

"Thank you, but I'm sure Mrs. Bromley only wants the dog to be all right."

With this I walked away and joined a distressed Mrs. Bromley. We waited for quite a while. I tried to comfort her, but she was devastated. She talked incessantly while I prayed to God to spare Bowdie's life and for Mrs. Bromley to have the strength to handle it should Bowdie die.

Finally, the veterinarian called us into the examining room. I was heartbroken to see Bowdie lying on a table, her two legs in casts. When she saw us, she tried to lift her head, and whimpered. Her little tail barely moved. Mrs. Bromley ran to her side.

"Baby, are you in pain? Oh, my little treasure, it breaks my heart to see you like this." She looked upward. "God, don't let her suffer. I rather be the one in pain."

"Doctor, is she going to be okay?" I asked.

"Her legs are crushed," he said somberly. "I wouldn't advise an operation. At her age she wouldn't make it."

"What did you say?" Mrs. Bromley asked.

He repeated what he had said.

"You don't know what you're talking about," she snapped. "Let's take Bowdie to her own doctor."

The doctor rearranged his glasses. "If that's your wish, I'll have the dog taken to your car. Be careful how you handle her."

We drove to the clinic. Luckily, the veterinarian took us to the examining room immediately. I handed him the X-rays the other doctor had given me. He looked at them and shook his head.

"What is it?" Mrs. Bromley asked, obviously distressed. "Tell me the truth."

"I'm afraid…not good news," he said. "I'm sorry, but Bowdie won't make it through the kind of operation needed."

"Money is not an issue," she argued. "Call the best surgeon, but please save my baby."

"Money has nothing to do with it. The dog is old and frail. Even if she survived the surgery, she'd be in excruciating pain. She wouldn't be able to go to the bathroom by herself; you'd have to hold her up with a towel. With this kind of life and lack of movement, she wouldn't last long anyway."

"What would you do if it were your dog?" I asked.

"Without a doubt, I'd put an end to her suffering."

Mrs. Bromley clutched my hand. "Lolita, what does he mean? What are we going to do?"

"We must be strong," I said, almost crying. "Our baby has no chance to recover, and she's in too much pain. We don't want her to suffer, do we? Look at her. She's pleading for help! Please, dear, don't let her suffer anymore."

"I don't want her to suffer." She sobbed. "Do what you need to do."

With a deep sigh, the vet said, "Mrs. Bromley, you made the right decision. Now, please wait outside while I prepare her. I'll call you when she's ready."

We sat outside and waited for what seemed an eternity. Mrs. Bromley couldn't stop crying. Finally the vet called us in. Bowdie lay on the table, with an IV attached to her. "You can stay with her as long as you wish. Once the needle is activated, it should only take a couple of seconds before she's gone."

After the doctor left, Mrs. Bromley caressed her dog. "My dear precious baby, I never thought you would go first."

Bowdie opened her eyes and closed them again, as if to say good-bye. I was on the verge of tears as Mrs. Bromley cradled her dear dog in her arms.

"Baby, I'm sorry I can't give you your life back. Thanks for the happiness you brought to my life. How am I going to survive without you?" She carefully raised Bowdie's face next to her own and sobbed.

Soon, Bowdie was going to be in dog heaven, if there was one, and Mrs. Bromley was going to need a lot of support and care. Concerned that she might suffer a heart attack, I called the vet, so he could proceed with the inevitable.

The doctor walked in and talked to Mrs. Bromley.

"My dear lady, the moment has come. You may leave now. Don't worry, I'll take care of everything else."

"I'm not moving from here until my baby's gone."

"I think it would be better for you to leave."

"Keep your advice to yourself. I'll be right here until the end."

"If that's what you wish." He proceeded to activate the IV.

In a matter of seconds, Bowdie was gone. Mrs. Bromley began to wail, and her body shook as she sank into a chair.

"Lolita, I'm all alone now." She wept. "Promise you will never leave me."

I sat next to her, enwrapped in a terrible feeling of powerless.

27

New Home

"Don't take my baby yet, doctor. Leave me alone with her." Mrs. Bromley clutched Bowdie's dead body. "Don't leave me alone, baby!" she cried.

"God, why did you do this to me? First Robert left me, and now my treasure. What am I going to do without her?"

She looked so devastated. My heart cried for her. Although we were bound by the same grief, she couldn't do anything to help me with my pain, but I could do a lot to lessen hers. Accepting a new job at a time like this would be like prodding deeper into her broken heart, and I wondered if I would have the heart to leave her. Her anguish made the lump in my throat tighten. I threw my arms around her, thinking that if I were to take the other job, this could be our last embrace.

From the depths of my heart, I said, "Dear Mrs. Bromley, I promise I'll take care of you for as long as you need me."

"Don't ever leave me, Lolita," she faltered.

Our eyes met: hers with a desperate plea for love and understanding; mine filled with empathy. She pressed her face against mine, and I realized that it was the first physical contact between us. It made my love for her grow deeper.

I didn't hear Jane and Mr. Williams entering the room. All of the sudden, they were in front of us and I couldn't remember ever being so happy to see any-one. My first impulse was to hug them, but instead, I stepped aside so they could comfort Mrs. Bromley.

"I'm so sorry," they both said.

"My baby is gone," Mrs. Bromley lamented as she gently stroked Bowdie's fur.

Jane leaned over and caressed the dog's head tenderly. "Oh, God, how terri-ble, I know how you must feel, Betty."

"Nobody knows how I feel. Just tell me how I am going to go on without my baby."

"Darling Grandmere," Mr. Williams said tenderly, "we'll help you, and you'll never be alone. Trust me."

"Gary, I want to take Baby with me."

Mr. Williams gave his grandmother a soft glance. "Sweetheart, let the doctor take care of Bowdie. He knows what to do."

"He didn't save her when she was dying—why would I trust him and leave my baby here? I want her in my backyard, so I can talk to her every day."

"Betty, there's no life in Bowdie," Jane said lovingly. "There's nothing anyone can do for her. Let the people here take care of her." Jane looked genuinely concerned, running her fingers through her mother-in-law's hair. "You look tired, darling. You need to rest."

Mrs. Bromley grabbed her chest. "I'm hurting. I want this pain to go away. I want to take Bowdie home. That's all I ask. Have pity on me."

"Grandmere, that's enough," Mr. Williams said firmly. "We can't do that."

"Lolita," she begged, "don't let them take our Bowdie from us. We have to take her home where she belongs."

I lowered my voice. "Mr. Williams, let me talk to her alone, please. I'll try to convince her."

"Lolita, do you know what you are doing?" Jane asked.

"Of course. By force she won't agree to anything. Do you remember when she drank the Pine-Sol? She didn't want to leave the house, and the paramedics had to tie her to the stretcher. I don't want anyone using force on her again. I'll find a way to persuade her to leave Bowdie here. I'll make up some story. Leave it to me."

"Whatever you do, make sure Bowdie is left here," Jane insisted.

"I know, Jane. That's the whole point," I said.

Mr. Williams held my hand. "Lolita, I trust you. I really appreciate what you're doing."

Mr. Williams looked gloomy and despondent, which compelled me to at least try to give him peace of mind. Brokenhearted, I relinquished to my longtime dream and voiced my decision: "Mr. Williams, I won't take the other job, I'll stay with her as long as she needs me. I hope this will help you."

His expression brightened. "Oh, Lolita, that means so much to me. I really appreciate your staying with her."

Jane cuddled her mother-in-law and kissed her on both cheeks. "Darling, we're leaving. I'll see you at home in a little bit. I love you."

After they left, I wasn't sure how to start the painful task of separating her from Bowdie.

"Mrs. Bromley," I began, "let's go to the other room."

"I don't want to leave Baby alone."

"She was a very proud dog. I'm sure Bowdie doesn't want to be seen lying down lifeless. Do you recall a long time ago, when the vet shaved her? She was very sad and hid from everyone until her coat came back. Let's make arrangements now to put her in a cozy, cushioned box and lay her to rest, then we can leave." Mrs. Bromley looked confused, so I took advantage of it and insisted, "I feel bad for our dear Bowdie because I'm sure she doesn't like to be seen looking this way. We don't want to annoy and embarrassed her any further, so we'd better leave."

"You're right," without a fight she agreed, to my surprise. "Tell the doctor to put her in a box, so we can take her with us, and I promise I won't peek. I only want her close to me."

I thought of asking for an empty sealed box, but if the box were light, she'd know it was empty. Now I was in a dilemma. I started to build up a plan as I walked for the door, hoping that she'd follow me. I was relieved when she did. The doctor appeared, and she addressed him.

"Doctor, we're taking my baby home."

"But your family wants her cremated," he said.

"It's my dog, and it's my decision to take her home."

I gabbed the veterinary's arm and pulled him aside with my back to Mrs. Bromley and said in a low voice, "Doctor, Give me a few minutes, I'll convince her to leave the dog here."

The doctor agreed.

Mrs. Bromley and I sat in the waiting room. We embraced and we sobbed. Finally, I promised we would pick up Bowdie the next day and put her to rest in the backyard, under her bedroom window.

"Why wait until tomorrow?" she asked.

"My dear, they have to embalm her, and that takes all night."

She believed me. I hoped that by tomorrow she would have forgotten my words. I hated misleading her, but I needed to in order to appease brokenhearted Mrs. Bromley the pain of leaving without Bowdie.

The next day, she looked for Bowdie all over the house. She was aware that something was wrong, but not that Bowdie was gone forever. She insisted that we go to the hospital to pick her up. She was hurting, and there was nothing I could do.

Time went by, but it didn't bring peace. It was unbearable to see Mrs. Bromley wandering about the house, calling for Bowdie.

One sunny day, I brought a tray with breakfast to her room. I placed the tray on a little table by the window and pulled the drapes open.

"What day is today?" she asked, without interest.

"Today is Sunday, and we're going to church," I said, helping her out of bed and into a robe.

"Are you going out?"

"We're going to church," I said crisply, accentuating the "we."

"You mean you're going to church."

"Remember, we go every Sunday to mass and to lunch? Today is Sunday, and we're going."

"The only thing I remember is that God is not listening to me. Why should I go to church? What I want is to die and see Robert and Bowdie."

It felt like a stab in my heart each time she cried out that she wanted to die.

"Mrs. Bromley, you know that God has a reason for everything he does. Now, be good, have your breakfast, and be ready to wear the new dress Jane brought yesterday."

Some vanity was left in her. Her face lit up for a moment, and she demanded, "Bring it to me right now."

I brought the outfit out.

"Don't waste time—help me to get dressed," she ordered, getting to her feet.

"As soon as you finish your breakfast, I will," I said, pretending authority.

"Since when do you give orders around here? Go away. I'll clean up all my holes and get dressed myself."

. *Wonderful,* I thought. *There's still fire in my dear Mrs. Bromley.* I made believe I had left and hid in the closet. She did a good job of washing and getting dressed. I wondered how much longer she would be able to do it alone.

She did look very pretty and dignified in the navy-blue suit, which brought out the beauty of her blue eyes and the snow-white of her thick hair.

According to my own philosophy, everything bad in life brings some good. Even for Alzheimer's victims' families, there is some infinitesimal good hiding somewhere. That was why I appreciated the chance to share with Mrs. Bromley each moment of lucidity left in her being. I poured my compassion over her. I said "I love you" over and over again, which is something that a sudden death deprives us of. If any of my family members were seriously sick, I would pray, hoping for health; but faced with Alzheimer's, I would extend my farewells and help them along each step of the lonely journey.

Many times I felt on the brink of losing my patience and I wanted to scream because she wouldn't stop asking about Bowdie. I started wishing I could fly somewhere and disappear.

Given the choice of losing my mind or saving it, I chose the latter. One day, in desperation, I thought of a scheme to try to ease her pain even if only momentarily.

"Mrs. Bromley, please come with me."

"Where?"

"To talk to Bowdie. Let's go outside."

"What?"

"Follow me. You'll be happy."

"I don't know what you are talking about. What's the matter with you?" she asked.

"We're going to visit Bowdie. She's resting in peace in our backyard."

"You'd better explain—and be specific."

"Our adorable Bowdie is buried there. We'll bring a pretty flower and talk to her. She's waiting for us."

Her face lit up. "Is she there? I don't remember anything. When did they bring her?"

We walked to a flowerbed and I picked a rose.

"She's been there for a while, but we haven't visited her. Now I think it would be good for you and Bowdie to talk to each other."

We walked over to a shady corner, where I had nestled a plaque with the inscription: *REST IN PEACE, BELOVED BOWDIE.*

"How come I never saw this? It's your fault because you didn't write a note to keep in my purse. Write it now, so I can remember and come here every day."

I was glad my idea had worked. "I'm sorry about that," I said. "I'll write a note immediately. This flower is for Bowdie."

She pulled a lawn chair next to the plaque, and began to talk. "Don't be afraid, Baby, you're not alone...I'm here. I brought you a rose. I miss you, Baby..."

Her words faded as I walked away, keeping her within my view. I was satisfied, because I had found a way to make her happy, even if only with an empty grave.

I had also fulfilled the promise I had made when Bowdie was killed, when I had promised that I would stay with Mrs. Bromley as long as she needed me. I glanced at her. She was smiling, and I heard bits and pieces of her conversation.

The morning breeze brought fragments like, "Bowdie, dear, I'll tell you every-thing." "You aren't cold, are you?" and "You'll be close to me always."

It was like coming back to life. Her reunion with Bowdie made her happy, and I felt that sometimes a lie was necessary to ease pain, even if only momen-tarily. In this case, the end justified the means.

Other lies came back to mind: lies I had thought were necessary for the stabil-ity of my marriage. Like a movie reel playing a film, I watched as memories flashed across the screen of my mind. I remembered how I had altered the truth to give fleeting moments of happiness to my children. Now, once more, I resorted to the same method on behalf of Mrs. Bromley.

I remembered one time when my daughter Olivia, who was prone to melan-choly, beamed happily because of my fabrication. Mrs. Bromley now and my daughter a long time ago had a taste of happiness only because of my made-up stories.

One of my husband's arbitrary rules was not to let our two girls mingle with boys. Olivia, at fourteen, was shy, with low self-esteem, so when she begged me to organize a party, I felt obliged to comply.

There was a fifteen-year-old boy she liked but could only see from a distance. The boy found out that we owned a Steinway, and he wanted to play it. Olivia invited him, but she wanted an audience. Since my husband played poker every Tuesday at a friend's house, I chose the following Tuesday for the party.

When the day arrived, I wanted to make sure the poker game was still on.

"Are you playing tonight?" I asked indifferently, without looking at him.

"Today's Tuesday, isn't it?" he answered sharply.

"What time will it be over?" I asked softly.

"Is anything going on that I should know about?"

I looked at him and smiled. "Is there anything wrong with chatting?"

"A silly way of making conversation, I might add."

That was to be the end of my questioning. I had learned to wrap my senses with grease, so his harshness slid down, leaving my soul untouched. I have, at least, confirmed that the poker game was on for that night. With my mind at ease, I proceeded with the preparations.

The party was from seven to ten. I was certain that there would be plenty of time to clear up after the party before Mauricio's arrival, since he usually got home around three in the morning.

At nine, the party was going well, and the young man excelled at the piano. Olivia became alive; her sparkling eyes made up for any consequences this subterfuge could bring. That had happened in Mexico long time ago. But right now, in the United States, while working for a British lady, I was creating a similar deception to obtain moments of happiness.

I reminisced some more about Olivia's party, more memories were dancing in my mind. Those past experiences didn't hurt, nor did they weigh on my conscience any more.

In the household, we had all been afraid of Mauricio, so when I saw the maid rushing toward me, I suspected something was very wrong.

"*Señora* Rimblas, Don Mauricio just drove up," she said.

"Don't open the gate yet. Give me a moment to think."

First I hid the boys in several closets and the girls waited in the studio. I asked the maid to bring Olivia's backpack and all the notebooks that she could find.

Customarily, and when in a good mood, before entering the house, Mauricio would talk and play with our collie in the yard. Tonight he was mad because the maid didn't open the gate immediately. He brushed the dog away and came into the house. I raced to him and placed a perfunctory kiss on his cheek, which he didn't return.

"Where are the children?" he asked dryly.

"Leti and James are upstairs, and Olivia's doing homework with friends in the studio."

"Friends? How come I didn't know anything about it?"

"They called," I tried to explain, "because the girls were doing a team project for school and wanted Olivia to join them. Since I couldn't find you to ask first, I invited them to come here instead."

"Always ask me first," he said with authority, "and make sure it doesn't happen again. Send Olivia up to see me, please. I'll be in my room."

I went to look for Olivia and delivered her father's command. Olivia looked at me with her big black eyes filled with fear. "I'm still in my party dress," she said. "I'm afraid."

"Just throw yourself in his arms and say you love him. Don't give him time to react." I knew Olivia was safe. Mauricio could be violent with anyone but his children.

I called one of the mother's and told her what had happened. "Please, Teresa, pick up the boys outside the gate and my chauffer will drive the girls to their houses."

Back in the present and still reflecting on my past, I realized the false foundation on which I had based my children's happiness at that time, and Mrs. Bromley's now.

28

Finale

I tried to get another schnauzer for Mrs. Bromley, but Jane was against it. I asked permission to take her back to Leverocks to see Bryan. It was not recommended. I wanted to take her to Cocoa Beach to visit Bill. Another negative. I was limited in my resources and forced to work with what I had to bring Mrs. Bromley back to her little pleasures. I asked Leti and Japhlet to give some of their time. They both were extremely busy; Leti with private classes, and Japhlet with after-school guitar lessons and homework. Nevertheless, they helped me. I couldn't find enough words to express my gratitude to them for bringing some joy into the fragile spirit of the grieving Mrs. Bromley.

On their first visit, Japhlet brought his guitar and amplifier. It pleased me that slowly Mrs. Bromley's expression softened while being serenaded. By the end, she was looking at him steadily with a sweet smile on her lips.

The following week, they took her on a boat ride around Boca Ciega Bay. Mrs. Bromley looked radiant upon their return home. Leti said Mrs. Bromley felt at home on the boat.

One Saturday afternoon, Leti had to meet with some teachers from her school, so Japhlet agreed to entertain Mrs. Bromley while I went to run some of my errands.

When I came back, Japhlet sat next to me and Leti helped Mrs. Bromley get ready for bed.

"*Abuelita*, do you want to hear what happened today with Mrs. Bromley?"

"Oh, yes. I want to know exactly what she said. Her behavior and her vocabulary are my yardstick to measure the progress of her illness. Tell me, word by word, as best as you remember."

"Okay. We went to an outside café not far from here. My mom and the teachers sat at one table, and I sat with Mrs. Bromley at another. We talked about the usual—you know, music, dancing, my hair, and when I was planning to cut it.

As it got late, she started getting more and more uneasy. 'What time is it?' she asked every five minutes. 'We should be heading home.'

"We have to wait. My mom is in a meeting," I told her. "Why don't we walk over to the dock?" 'I don't want to. Just be a darling and order me a glass of wine,' she said, with her cute smile.

"They don't serve wine here; it's a coffee shop," I said. "Besides, I am under-age. I can't order wine for you."

'Oh, how boring. That is not fun at all.' She frowned and glanced around nervously."

'You can have some of my scotch when we get home,' she insisted in a low voice and a cute smile. *Abuelita*, at that she got up and started walking away. I followed her to a liquor store and waited outside. She finally came out with what I later found out was a small bottle of scotch. When she got back to the table, she started sipping out of the bottle with the paper bag around it and all."

'Would you like some, Danny?' she asked.

'I can't drink yet, Mrs. Bromley. I'm sixteen.'

'Sixteen? And your mother won't let you drink?'

'It's not that my mother won't let me. But I'm a minor and it's against the law.'

'All right, you are right.'

Japhlet shrugged. "She didn't bug me about the time any more and my mom was able to finish her meeting without a scene," he exclaimed triumphantly.

"It sounds like Mrs. Bromley is still with us. I'm so glad you helped to shake her out of her idleness. It's not all lost—not yet, anyway."

Once Mrs. Bromley was in bed they left with my blessings.

The following months, Mrs. Bromley got her *third* wind, but It was necessary for my children to cut their visits considerably. In my desire to entertain her and keep her brain working, I brought Maurice Chevalier's film *The Merry Widow*, thinking that she would be delighted. She wasn't able to sit for long, she jumped to her feet and said, "In the past, he plummeted me into boredom, and now he almost killed me. He has not changed."

This woman never ceased to amaze me. She used almost the same words she used the first time she told me about her romance with Chevalier.

Days went by with more of the same. Mrs. Bromley's depression accentuated, and on many a day she refused to get out of bed, with the exception of her day in the beauty parlor when she didn't need much persuasion. She stopped enjoying her usual shopping sprees because Jane took away the checkbook. There was a constant argument about this but to my relief she blamed her family, not me. I was embarrassed to hear her ranting and raving each time we went to the bank to cash the checks, that as her family ordered, she signed but I wrote.

Every day, she made me look around for a brooch that Robert had given her on his deathbed. The brooch was an American flag made out of rubies and white and blue diamonds. Since she misplaced or threw away many valuables, Jane had opted to lock them in the bank. It broke my heart to watch her desperately trying to find the things she was so attached to. The one that pained her the most was the flag. Again, there was nothing I could do. Thinking of it now, we should have made a copy of the flag brooch, since it meant so much to her. But it was too late when I thought of that. I regretted it very much. My daily tasks were to look for her brooch and to look for her dog. In addition to that, there were occasional bathroom accidents. Even with my love for her and my optimistic outlook on life, I needed a rest from this in order to come back full of energy again. I was frustrated and on the verge of a breakdown. I urgently needed to recharge my batteries so I could keep giving her my best.

I voiced my concerns to my daughter Olivia, and she persuaded me to go visit them. To go on without a break would work against Mrs. Bromley, because if I got fed up, she would suffer the consequences. I made reservations to go to Minnesota.

Mr. Williams, as always, supported me and gave me his blessing. I spoke to Meri, and she agreed to help out. Jane offered to find a woman to bathe Mrs. Bromley. She said not to worry; she'll look after her mother-in-law. But my heart was heavy with worry. I decided to brush away a premonition hovering over me. Remorse played its part in my feelings and I almost decided against my trip.

The day of my departure arrived. I left very happy because I was going to see my daughter Olivia and my son, James, as well as my grandchildren. But I was carrying a heavy burden because I was leaving difficult Mrs. Bromley.

I was happy to visit my family, and the beautiful June weather in Minneapolis soothed me. I didn't call Mrs. Bromley right away, because I was afraid of hearing bad news, which would ruin my stay. After a few great days with my family, my good spirits already renewed, I called Mrs. Bromley's house, but there was no answer. I tried the next day in the morning and in the evening. When no one answered the phone, I called Jane.

After we greeted one another, I asked about Mrs. Bromley. She came right to the point.

"I placed her in a home. A very nice one."

I felt as if icy water were rushing through my body. I swallowed the first words that came to mind. With a chill running down my spine, I asked, refraining from yelling, "Why did you do that? Why didn't you call me first?"

"I didn't want to spoil your visit with your family."

I was angered by the absurd excuse she had given me.

"What prompted you to do such a thing?" I asked in disbelief.

"She got very aggressive and wanted Meri to dig Bowdie out of the ground."

"I should have taken the plaque away before I left."

"Yes, you should have. But things happened for the best. Betty's happy there, and they know how to handle her. Now we all have peace of mind."

There was silence, which she broke. "Don't worry. We'll compensate you gladly. Take your time with your children, and when you come back, we'll take Betty to lunch. She's confused, and sometimes she doesn't remember me."

Of course she's confused after being ripped out of her accustomed surroundings and away from her belongings. It's inhuman. I felt like screaming.

"I hope you're right and that this is best for her," I said, and hung up the phone.

I was terribly upset, but I realized that I wasn't family. It was sad that sentimental bonds didn't count; otherwise they would have taken my feelings into consideration. No one had spent more time and invested more energy on Mrs. Bromley than I, but after all, it was an important family decision, and who was I to be included? I wanted urgently to bring a little peace to my heart, but the sad truth was that I had been cut off from Mrs. Bromley's life, and it hurt beyond belief.

There was a knot in my stomach. Besides the emptiness I felt for myself and for Mrs. Bromley, I had another headache to contend with: how would I pay my mortgage? The only solution I could think of—and dreaded—was to sell my cherished home. I also regretted enormously the loss of my lifelong dream, to which I renounced for the well-being of Mr. Williams and Mrs. Bromley—there was no use in complaining—now it was beyond reproach, and what was worse, beyond repair.

I extended the stay with my children, and when I finally returned to Florida, I went to visit Mrs. Bromley. Jane made the arrangements, and we took her out to lunch. I was heartbroken to see how much she had changed in little over two months. I saw a shell of who she used to be, finally giving way to old age, oblivious to her surroundings and depleted of life. Where was my spirited and proud Mrs. Bromley? My heart cried for her, but I struggled to hide my ache.

"Hello, Mrs. Bromley. I'm Lolita," I said, holding her cold hands. "Do you remember me?"

She shook her head many times, scanning the room as if afraid of something.

Jane explained, "Betty, Lolita was your companion for years. You both got along fabulously. Remember?"

There was an empty look from Mrs. Bromley, and again she shook her head.

"We're taking you to lunch," Jane added. "Would you like that?"

She nodded, with the same empty look that broke my heart.

"The disease suddenly advanced very rapidly," Jane whispered. "She's not talking anymore."

Once we were seated in the restaurant, I held Mrs. Bromley's hand for a long time, searching her expression for a sign that she remembered me. After all, I was the person who for years kept her company day and night. I hoped that a spark of consciousness was hidden somewhere.

"Do you remember Bowdie?" I asked. "We used to take her to the park near your house. Remember we went to a different restaurant every day and to the bank? You loved to write checks, go grocery shopping, and go to the mall. You bought tons of beauty supplies. We sure had good times together." Her expression did not change, although her blank gaze was fixed on me. The waitress came to our table, ready to take our order.

"Jane," I said, "please order for us. You know what she likes. Get the same for me." As soon as the waitress left with our order, I quickly turned my attention back to Mrs. Bromley and squeezed her hand tenderly. "You enjoyed going to church with me, remember?" I asked softly. "We went to mass every Sunday, but you wanted to go every day. First thing in the morning, you'd stand by my door and chant 'I'm ready. Where's Lolita? I don't like to wait. I'm ready.'"

Suddenly, I saw it. *Almighty God!* I could hardly believe it, but I saw a ray of light in her eyes; there was life in her. Something I had said must have triggered a cord in her memory, encouraging me to continue. "Remember the zoo, when you spoke with the giraffe? Do you remember Danny, the young boy with long hair and a guitar? His mother's name is Leti, and you liked them a lot. In fact, you preferred them over me. They took you everywhere."

When the waitress came with the food, Jane placed it very gingerly in front of us and motioned for the waitress to leave. Then Jane helped Mrs. Bromley with the soup. Mrs. Bromley held the glass of wine herself. With her eyes, Mrs. Bromley followed my every movement carefully. I ate very quickly. I didn't want to lose momentum; I wanted to go on with my conversation.

I saw a shadow of a smile on her face and repressed the impulse to take her in my arms in the tight embrace she had repelled so many times. Rapidly, I returned all my attention to her and continued, slowly, clearly enunciating every word. "Do you remember when you visited my daughter's school and the children interviewed you? You gave a gift to each one, and then I took pictures of you with the kids. Remember? And they showed you their pet snake. You love animals.

You and I made quite a team. We share good memories, you and I."

I sipped some of my wine, and her eyes followed me. Her face was no longer expressionless. I couldn't figure out what kind of expression it was, but there was one. This fueled me to keep on prying, trying to bring her into some form of consciousness.

"Remember that we spent many nights looking at your newspaper clippings? The good reviews in the European papers? They brought you wonderful memories. And how many hours we talked about your dancing days! You had a romance with Maurice Chevalier! He sent flowers to your dressing room every day. Oh, gosh—your sister Zinna and her friendship with the queen of Spain? You must remember that." Remember we play-acted? We dressed up for the occasion."

Back at the nursing home, Mrs. Bromley walked straight to her bed, removed the stuffed animals, flung the pillows aside, and turned to Jane. "Ask Lolita to stay for a nap. The bed is ready for her."

I was flabbergasted. Mrs. Bromley had recognized me at last. This time I couldn't repress my need to hug her, and I pulled her into my arms in an embrace close to my heart, wishing to transmit my love and compassion with the human touch she needed so much. Her brief moment of lucidity boggled my mind. I stayed for a little longer, and when I kissed her good-bye, the sadness in her expression filled my heart with tears. I knew I was going to remember the emptiness in her eyes all my life, and the sadness in her expression would haunt me forever.

The next day, Jane called to inform me that when Mrs. Bromley had gotten up, she dressed without help, and announced, "I'm ready for church. Where are my gloves? I don't like to wait. Where is Lolita?"

The End

Epilogue

I sat on my favorite rattan rocking chair in the front porch of *my* house with a relaxed half smile on my face. I listened to the seagulls squall as they flew by to the beach across from me. I reflected on all that had happened since I last saw Mrs. Bromley. My heart ached for her, but I felt immense satisfaction knowing that I had made a difference in her life. I knew that the inevitable devastation brought by Alzheimer's could not be halted and I also knew that the path to the end could be less painful with love, caring and patience. I had hoped to be with her until the end, to hold her hand and pray until her spirit transcended beyond the finite—free at last; but to do so was not in my control.

I closed my eyes trying to catch a midday nap, but another revealing thought crept into my mind as I realized that I felt better about myself than ever before. It was true that I was packing my belongings to leave *my* house forever, because without a job I had no way to pay the mortgage. Surprisingly, I no longer had the need to hold onto the house.

I remembered Ralph Emerson's philosophy that you lose something to gain something more valuable. I had health, the care of a loving family and the capacity to create new memories. I'll use my time to write the book I have dancing in my head about the memorable character that changed the way I saw life. I couldn't wait to put it down in words.

I settled back on my rocking chair for a little longer. Leti and Japhlet were helping me move. The bank was repossessing the house and we were going to drive to Minnesota where I was to live with my daughter Olivia.

I started to get up when I felt Leti's hand softly rest on my shoulder as the other hand caressed my hair, with a kiss on my forehead she asked, "Are you okay, mamita?"

"Yes, honey, I'm fine."

"Abuelita, are you going to miss the beach?" asked Japhlet playfully. He seemed so carefree lately—such a joy to watch.

"Come to think of it...I don't think so. I'll be very busy experiencing the change of seasons and Minnesota's 10,000 lakes," I said, meaning it.

"I just need to finish this last box and we can go," Leti announced.

Once we were packed and ready to leave, I walked out of *my* house for the last time and into a new and very different life.

978-0-595-37351-2
0-595-37351-8